CBD Oil for Pain Relief

How to get Healthy without
Prescription Medications

By Charles Coles

Table of Contents

Introduction

The following chapters will discuss the effects and uses of CBD on various diseases, as well as information on what it is and obtaining it, among other things. It often gets a bad reputation due to the stigma of being associated with marijuana, which will also be covered in these chapters.

I wanted to write this book because CBD has been greatly important to my life and well-being. When I was a teen, I was diagnosed with fibromyalgia, a chronic and lifelong muscle pain that prescription medications were never able to truly help with. I tried many treatments, all with little to no long term success. I majored in Biology in college, going so far as to pick up a minor in Health Sciences to possibly learn more about my own condition, and faced few results there as well.

Finally, a friend pointed me in the direction of CBD oil, and the outcome was life changing. My pain was more manageable than ever before, and I became intrigued by something so beneficial that is so relatively unknown to the general public. I began to do research, both on CBD and on its affects with a range of mental and physical problems, and have compiled it all here for you. This has been an important project for me, since something so beneficial shouldn't be as hard to access and as stigmatized as it is.

By spreading proper education and research, we can help to end this stigma one person at a time. I would also like for this to be helpful for those with their own pains, so they can learn how to try CBD safely and effectively for themselves, having to do less guesswork than I did. By taking some of the frustration out of the process, the right results are more achievable.

There are plenty of books on this subject on the market, so thank you again for choosing this one! Every effort was made to ensure it is full of as much useful information, research, and facts as possible, please enjoy!

Chapter 1

An Introduction to
CBD

Welcome to the ever expanding world of cannabis, and congratulations on checking out the benefits of CBD (also known as cannabidiol) oil for yourself.

People all over the world have had a long standing relationship with marijuana and hemp, dating back thousands of years and covering a wide variety of uses. The Chinese called it "the plant of a thousand uses," and rightly so. Medical marijuana dates back as far as B.C. times, when the Chinese used it to treat conditions such as inflammation and uterus pains.

There is an impressive record throughout history (until the recent 20th century that is) of the marijuana plant contributing in many ways to medical conditions. One of the more recent contributions from hemp to society, though, has been CBD oil.

To begin, one of the most often asked questions regarding CBD: what is it, and how is it different from traditional marijuana (THC)? CBD is a naturally occurring extract in either powder form or oil that can be taken from both marijuana plants and hemp plants, which, while similar, in fact have slightly different genetic makeups.

Hemp is ideal for CBD extraction, as it typically contains much lower amounts of tetrahydrocannabinol (THC) which is the actual compound that causes the psychoactive effect in the brain, or getting 'high.' This makes it an ideal treatment for those who have no interest in those highs, who regularly get drug tested, or are children, the elderly, or anybody else that may want to stay away from regular weed. In this book, we will focus specifically on CBD and its up and coming potential to help an incredible range of diseases.

CBD has been shown to help with many issues, including but not limited to:

- Pain relief
- Anxiety relief
- Seizure prevention
- Insomnia prevention

- Heart health
- Clearer skin
- Memory
- Inflammation

It is suspected to be able to do all of this by acting on the endocannabinoid system, including two receptors called CB1 and CB2, which help the body regulate its systems for sleep, digestion, immunity, memory, and pleasure reception, among many other things. In fact, the endocannabinoid system was discovered and named *after* cannabis, further demonstrating the usefulness of this plant upon people. It effectively helps neutralize the system, preventing it from heading towards one extreme or another, and keeps the body in a sort of balance, also known as homeostasis.

There are two main types of these endocannabinoid receptors in the body that CBD acts on: CB1 and CB2. CB1 is associated with the central nervous system, while CB2 affects the body's immunity and intestines. Between the two, there is very little in the human body that CBD can't help or come into contact with.

It increases the amount of endocannabinoids in your system, helping your body to effectively heal, balance and regulate itself. This has been shown to possibly able to do things that prescription medications simply can't (at least, not without major side effects): reverse nerve damage, lower inflammation, reduce anxiety, and more.

CBD comes in a variety of products and methods of ingestion. One of the most popular and well-known is the tincture, or dropper, which allows the CBD to be placed directly under your tongue. This is also one of the quickest and most efficient methods of ingestion, since it allows the CBD to be absorbed by the body in as little as 15 minutes. Other popular ones include vaping, capsules, edibles (including cooking it into a variety of foods), and powder form.

CBD oil has only been around for a few decades, but it is already making ripples and waves in the medical community. There has been major headway made for it as a more effective medicine than traditional prescription meds against diseases like epilepsy and anxiety, and there are more studies coming out every year.

The cannabis community as a whole is growing louder every year and pushing for full federal government legalization, and cannot be ignored for much longer. Changes are already beginning to show as new marijuana friendly laws begin to appear on ballots nationwide during election times.

CBD can be, unlike traditional western medicine, almost a fully self-sufficient customer product. Once you have done your research, learned what it takes to work for you, and adjusted your dosages to your needs, you can even make it for yourself. No other medication allows for this, and the freedom to take care of your own needs is a luxury that is both satisfying and cost reducing, especially in the face of today's incredibly expensive healthcare system.

Personally, I have struggled with health problems for all of my adult life. The constant doctor visits, the useless lab tests, the lack of help from prescription medications—it all built up over the years to an incredible amount of frustration and had a major effect on my overall quality of life.

Even with my diagnosis of fibromyalgia, I had a hard time getting doctors to truly provide help to reduce my pain and often felt as though my lab test results were disregarded. I was fortunate enough to have a friend recommend CBD oil to me, and the results were life changing. I felt such a drastic increase in my daily health and happiness that it drove me to do the research seen here, and hopefully help others with their quality of life, as well.

In this book, we will cover a variety of topics regarding CBD: strains, doses, how it reacts and treats a number of diseases and ailments, and even animal use for your beloved furry friends and pets. I would like for this to serve as a guide to you as you begin your CBD journey and learn about all the cannabis world has to offer!

Before we begin however, a word of caution; while beneficial and low-risk, CBD is still a relatively new product that can come with side effects and from untrustworthy sources. Hemp derives a lot of nutrients from the ground, and growers who use pesticides can have those harmful chemicals end up in their CBD, among other things. Before taking this for yourself, talk to your primary physician or doctor, especially if you are already taking prescription medications, as CBD can interact with some of the same enzymes and may cause unexpected results.

Be cautious when starting out and frugal with your dosages to avoid any unwanted side effects or other problems, and make sure that the particular symptoms you would like to treat are in fact benefited by CBD oil. This part shouldn't be difficult, since the range of conditions shown to be helped by CBD only continue to grow, and where clinical trials lack, patient testimonials often come in.

Let's get started!

• Chapter 2 •

The history of
CBD

When many people think of CBD oil, they think of the cannabis plant, and rightly so. The cannabis plant itself has been used across many cultures, all the way back to ancient times. Everyone from the Chinese, to the Vikings, to Arabian people used it for a wide variety of things such as an addition to food, hemp, and paper.

There has even been some evidence that cavemen may have burned large piles of marijuana plants for the relaxing smoke effects. While THC and hemp was in widespread use for much of humanity, CBD oil only truly dates back to the 1940s, when it was first extracted from the cannabis plant by a scientist named Roger Adams.

THC and marijuana use has been around for centuries, but this is the first recorded and known interaction with specifically CBD itself. Like many other drugs, it was initially tested on small animals such as mice, beginning only a few years after its discovery. The original experiments were often done to compare CBD to THC, and proved that the physical effects of CBD didn't cause the same behavioral changes that THC did.

It wasn't until the 60s, though, that the actual compounds were discovered, and scientists figured out the real difference between the two. This was an important breakthrough within the cannabis community, since this provided an entirely new side of potential medicinal uses without the worry of getting high, which ruled out THC treatments for many patients.

From there, the excitement and interest for medicinal use only grew. In the 70s, it began to break ground as a legitimate and useable treatment, becoming legally recognized by New Mexico in 1978. While there was still a ways to go before becoming fully legal, this was a forward step for CBD. The 80's also saw quite a bit of progress, with the first trials of CBD as a treatment for epilepsy.

Dr. Raphael Mechoulam, who'd been studying CBD since the 1960s, headed these trials with a team of researchers to determine the effectiveness of the oil, and had roaring success. All of the 16 patients they tested on had drastic results, which should have been a major turning point for the medicinal use of CBD oil. (More details on this case study can be found in Chapter 11).

Unfortunately, the United States was well underway with marijuana prohibition by this point, and the results garnered little attention from the medical field or the population as a whole. This was disappointing for these researchers, as the results should have spoken for themselves. However, there would be little other progress until 1996, when California became the first state to legalize medicinal marijuana. This was the beginning of the destigmatizing of marijuana and the cannabis plant as a whole, which would bode well for CBD.

Since those initial trials, the majority of growth surrounding the use of CBD as a product has come after 2000. In 2014, it was legalized for medicinal use in Alabama, Florida, Iowa, Kentucky, Mississippi, Missouri, North Carolina, South

Carolina, Tennessee, Utah, and Wisconsin. By the time of this book's publication, it's been legalized for medicinal use in 46 states, and legalized for recreational use (alongside marijuana) in 8.

Past this point, the laws and legislation get quite murky, but if a person is dedicated to the use of it is no longer nearly as hard to obtain. The major advancement of the marijuana plant and industry in the last decade has come with major steps forward for CBD users, and it's easier than ever before to access.

The marijuana industry has faced a lot of backlash and negativity over the last decades. Its classification as a Schedule I drug (considered the same level of dangerous and addictive as heroin and cocaine) have made it difficult to get any sort of federal regulation passed. It wasn't always this way—back in the 19th century, marijuana and cannabis-infused products were easy to find in drugstores as medicine for several different ailments.

It was the eventual Alcohol Prohibition, and later the War on Drugs, that heavily slowed down progress. American citizens, however, are taking it upon themselves to change this on state levels and hopefully, in the future, on the federal level. Additionally, another great helper to the marijuana industry has been college students.

While the college youth of today are often viewed as alcoholics freely attending fraternity parties, in the 1960s they were viewed with much more distinction, often the sons and daughters of the much wealthier upper class families, and when they took to smoking marijuana few were eager to lock them all up.

This spread from those original flower children on down, and changed the face of American drug culture forever. The damage done by the prohibition is slowly being reversed, and the newer, younger generations are much more marijuana-friendly than their parents, for many reasons.

Much of the history involving CBD is still unwritten, since there is clearly still a lot of progress to be made. The industry is hopeful for the day when CBD, and other medical marijuana products, can be prescribed by a doctor like other pharmaceuticals, allowing it to reach a whole new clientele that may be less afraid of the surrounding stigma. As studies and the benefits continue to come out, we will continue to push forward for that day, secure in the knowledge that cannabis has truly been a giving plant all along.

A summarized timeline of CBD oil thus far:

- 1940- CBD first extracted from cannabis plant. At the time, nobody was quite sure what it was or how to differentiate it between THC
- 1946- first CBD tests on lab animals, demonstrated no psychoactive effects
- 1946- CBD's three dimensional structure discovered
- 1964- This same compound was described in more depth, and differentiated between THC

- 1960s- lab tests on animals continued, proof of non-psychoactive effects confirmed
- 1970s- British Pharmacopoeia listed CBD as a potential medicine
- 1978- New Mexico acknowledges cannabis as medicine
- 1980- first major study on CBD run by Dr. Raphael Mechoulam conducted on epilepsy, showed shockingly promising results
- 1996- California becomes first state to legalize medical marijuana
- 2013- the widely publicized case of Charlotte Figi breaks
- 2014- legalization of CBD for medicinal use in 11 states

- Chapter 3 -

Legality

When it comes to CBD, one of the most murky and confusing aspects of it boils down to the simple question: where is it and where is it not legal?

This is made even more confusing when considering that state governments and federal governments do not always operate under the same system, and often do not follow the same laws. For example, while it is completely legal to smoke recreational marijuana in states like Colorado and California, you can still be prosecuted for smoking in national parks in those states, due to the government that maintains and runs them. Since those national parks are federal, and not state-operated, you can be busted, since recreational smoking is still highly illegal on the federal level.

In fact, the United States government is extremely anti-cannabis. Marijuana and its constituents are still classified as Schedule I drugs, and a lot of law enforcement is dedicated to prosecuting those who possess, sell, and use any cannabis related products, as well as cannabis itself. In fact, there have been more than 12 million marijuana related arrests since 1995, with someone being arrested for a cannabis related crime every minute.

These numbers are astronomical for a product that the majority of American citizens (a whopping 61 percent) want cannabis legalized, whether it be for medical purposes or purely recreational. The demand is there, and it cannot be ignored for much longer.

CBD has slightly more lenient, but also more complicated, laws than regular old marijuana. Since there are no psychoactive effects, many more states have approved it for varying uses. The 29 states in which it is legal for medical purposes with no restrictions on the production of the CBD include:

- Alaska
- Arizona
- Arkansas
- California
- Colorado

- Connecticut
- Delaware
- Florida
- Hawaii
- Illinois
- Maine
- Maryland
- Massachusetts
- Michigan
- Minnesota
- Montana
- Nevada
- New Hampshire
- New Jersey
- New Mexico
- New York
- North Dakota
- Ohio
- Oregon
- Pennsylvania
- Rhode Island
- Vermont
- Washington
- West Virginia

A prescription is required to get CBD in these states, except for the 9 in which all marijuana products are fully legalized. There are also restrictions in each state on the amount of THC allowed to be in CBD products, which varies by state. As for the rest of the US, there are a handful more states that also have laws about the legality of CBD, and permit it for medical use but require specific things regarding the treatment and production of the CBD, as well as restrictions on which medical conditions CBD can be used for. These states include:

- Alabama
- Florida
- Georgia
- Indiana
- Iowa
- Kentucky
- Mississippi
- Missouri
- North Carolina
- Oklahoma
- South Carolina

- Tennessee
- Texas
- Utah
- Virginia
- Wisconsin
- Wyoming

The remaining four states (Kansas, Nebraska, Idaho, and South Dakota) have far murkier laws regarding CBD. It is virtually illegal in these states, although both Nebraska and Idaho may have plans to change this soon.

Another factor in the legalization of CBD to consider is the cases currently, or in the past, being fought against both the federal government and the DEA to make these changes. One such case just ended in May of 2018, and those fighting for the side of CBD unfortunately lost. It originally began in 2016 when the DEA attempted to argue for the continued unlawfulness of CBD, due to the fact that it can come from the marijuana plant.

This was a shock to many, and outraged quite a few, who argued back that CBD can also be derived from hemp. While setbacks like this are common and often in the entire marijuana industry, it should not serve as a deterrent to those who are adamant about its benefits and eventual legalization.

Some laws that have been passed do not technically "allow" for CBD, but they do not persecute the possession of it. One of the more well-known examples of this is "Carly's Law" in Alabama, which was passed in 2014 and decriminalized the possession of CBD for the use of epileptic disorders. While this only allows it specifically for epilepsy and cannot be prescribed, but 'recommended,' it was still considered a step forward for CBD users within the state, and a testament to the usefulness of CBD against epilepsy.

The most important thing to consider before buying CBD in your state is to keep in mind that laws are subject to change, and every state has slightly different THC levels and specific clauses that other states don't have.

I advise anyone interested in getting CBD products for themselves to do some research on your current states' laws, especially since so many of them still require a prescription from a licensed physician. Every year, more states push cannabis-friendly legislature forward, and with any luck medical marijuana and CBD will be freely legal across the entire United States.

Chapter 4

Making your own
CBD

If you use high amounts of CBD oil on a regular basis, you just may benefit from growing, creating or cultivating it by yourself. It is a lot simpler and less complicated than it may seem, and there are a couple of ways to do it depending on whether you are extracting it from marijuana or from hemp.

Before we get into how to make it, though, we should look at a couple of other factors: namely, safety and legality. There are always safety precautions to take before doing anything you are planning to ingest and store for long term use. And of course, depending on your state, it may not be legal to either possess the marijuana to make it or to cultivate your own.

Safety

The actual process of making CBD oil is relatively safe, but there are things you can do to be sure you come out with the best possible product. Of course, make sure all jars/utensils/strainers/pans are as clean as possible and free of any residue such as dust or food. You are going to want airtight containers free of imperfections such as cracks or leaks. Some of the processes to make CBD involve using heat, either from the oven or stove, so be sure to use caution here as well, as any kind of oil can burn when heated.

One of the most important safety concerns is to be sure the product itself is as pure and clean as possible. You want to be certain you know both the strain and amount of CBD and THC in the marijuana or hemp you are deriving your CBD from, so you can know exactly what you are ending up with.

One way to make sure of this is to either know the grower you are purchasing from personally, to grow it yourself, or to do thorough research on any hemp/marijuana and the person or company selling it before you buy. You want to make sure your plants are GMO and pesticide free, as well as contaminant free.

Along with buying the purest and cleanest possible product, there are also a few strains of marijuana and hemp that are ideal for CBD extraction. A few of these include Charlotte's Web, Harlequin, Sour Tsunami, and Cannatonic.

Legality

We have covered the legal status of CBD itself, but what about making your own? Unfortunately, the laws there tend to be just as complicated as the laws about buying and using it. In any state where medical and recreational marijuana is completely legal, congratulations! You are free to make your own CBD to your heart's content, as long as you do not sell it without the proper licensure.

If you do not live in a marijuana-free state, the best way to avoid any kind of legal trouble is to research the laws within your state regarding possession, and absolutely do not attempt to sell CBD oil to others without first getting proper licenses, which may not even be available in your state. If you are only making CBD for yourself, in most states this should not be an issue if it is derived from hemp, but if you still live in a state where marijuana is completely illegal, you may encounter more roadblocks.

There are several different ways to make your own CBD oil. This first one infuses CBD from low THC strains of marijuana into another type of oil such as coconut, almond, or olive oil. This can be used for cooking or as a topical skin salve.

- **Step One:** Spread out the marijuana buds onto a flat cooking sheet, and bake in the oven at 200 degrees for about an hour. This is called decarboxylation.
- **Step Two:** Move the cooked buds into a jar, and completely cover them in one of the above oils of your choice. There should be standing liquid in the jar!
- **Step Three:** Store in a dark place for 4-6 weeks.
- **Step Four:** Strain the oil through a very fine sieve, or even a nylon stocking, into a new, clean jar. You can do some squeezing and

manipulating to get as much of the oil out as possible.

And that's it! You now have a CBD infused oil for whatever you would like to do with it. This process is ideal for those who want something extremely simple and have some time on their hands to wait.

The next process involves extracting CBD from hemp itself, which makes for both higher CBD content and is much more legally safe. It is very similar to the previous process and will also extract the CBD into an oil such as olive or coconut, so keep this in mind. This will also make the CBD perishable, and it should be stored in a cool, dark place after extraction.

- **Step One:** Place raw hemp materials on a flat cooking sheet and bake in the oven at 200 degrees Fahrenheit for 1 hour.
- **Step Two:** Add the plant material to a jar and fill with your choice of olive or coconut oils. Seal the jar with a lid.

- **Step Three:** Place the jar inside a large pot on top of a washrag and fill the pot with a few inches of water. Put lid on the pot. Place on a stove and bring the water to a boil.
- **Step Four:** Leave on the stove for 1-2 hours, adding water as it evaporates.
- **Step Five:** Strain the oil through a sieve or cloth into an airtight glass container. That's it!

The final method we will go over for at home extraction creates pure CBD oil, instead of that infused with other oils. For this one you will want a small, clean glass jar with a dropper lid to place the CBD into after extraction.

- **Step One:** Place your cannabis buds into a bowl and cover completely with alcohol. Stir consistently for about five minutes.
- **Step Two:** Filter the alcohol through a strainer or sieve into a container such as a glass jar. You can repeat these first two steps if you want extra concentrated CBD.

- **Step Three:** Put the liquid into a double boiler and heat until it bubbles. Leave on a low heat and stir until the alcohol has completely evaporated.

- **Step Four:** Once the alcohol is gone, remove the remaining oil and place it into airtight containers BEFORE it completely cools. Once it is cooled it will harden some and be much more difficult to work with.

- **Step Five:** Keep stored in a cool, dark place. This concentrated CBD oil is completely safe for any use you would like it for.

These three relatively simple processes should help you with any at home CBD needs you desire. With some time and practice, you can become an expert in not only treating yourself with CBD, but also in creating it. By following the proper steps, this will only serve you better on your CBD journey and allow you complete freedom to know your CBD products are in fact pure and safe for your consumption, as well as saving you quite a bit of money on costly CBD oil.

Chapter 5

Precautions and Negative Side Effects

While CBD comes with far less side effects than traditional prescription medications and treatments, there are of course still things to watch out for and be aware of.

One of these involves the overall cannabis community. Since so much of it is still not regulated by the Food and Drug Administration (FDA) there is still quite a lot of 'sketchy' products on the market, both in stores and online. It is extremely advised to be cautious when purchasing CBD and to look carefully at both the ingredients and the CBD content, since there are no laws regulating distributors to either of these qualities. While much of the cannabis community is made of good people with good intentions, there are always the scammers to watch out for.

These untrustworthy vendors can scam and rip you off in a few different ways. One of these is by advertising their products as the cheapest. Like many other things in the world, it is advisable to avoid the cheapest oils you can find.

Pure CBD oil is pretty expensive to make in bulk, and if it is super inexpensive then it is likely that the sellers have skimped somewhere, whether it be on actual CBD content or by cutting corners on the process itself. Do a bit of research on the vendor you are interested in before you purchase.

There are many reputable sellers (and disreputable ones) on the internet to choose from, and choosing the right CBD oil can make all the difference between treating an ailment and losing money to get no results whatsoever. This is not the place to skimp and cut corners—a bad product will provide no help, and may cause you to lose your faith in CBD altogether!

To get you started, here are a few tips for buying CBD oil:

- Read customer reviews and ratings—often people will leave good recommendations if they have liked the product, and if you cannot find any reviews at all, that's probably a good sign to steer clear.

- Check the ingredients—pure CBD oil does not need any other ingredients. If it has been diluted with all sorts of other chemicals, stay away.
- See how long the company has been around. If they have been selling products for at least a few years, they are likely to be more trustworthy.
- If you can find out what strain of marijuana or hemp they are producing their CBD from (and most websites have a Q&A section where they will tell you this), you can be surer of the CBD and THC contents.

If you are purchasing your CBD from a physical store, it is still vital to check the ingredients, brand, and CBD content. Do not be afraid to ask the seller for help—it's their job to know, and if they can't help you pick out a good CBD oil, don't be afraid to take your business elsewhere.

The next thing to keep in mind when trying CBD oil is of course the potential for negative side effects. As we have already discussed, CBD comes with relatively few side effects, and there is no risk for death or comas or anything particularly nasty along those lines. However, through the clinical trials and studies that have been done thus far, doctors and scientists have reported a few recurring ones:

- Drowsiness
- Diarrhea
- Weight gain/loss
- Appetite increase/decrease
- Dry mouth
- Nausea

These symptoms are almost never present in people who have taken doses smaller than about 600mg, and none of them are life threatening, but can at the least be uncomfortable and inconvenient. CBD has also been known to interact with other traditional prescription drugs. It is metabolized and interacts with some of the same enzymes as other medications, such as clarithromycin, which is used to treat infections.

Because of this, if you are receiving any prescription medications it is extremely important to consult your doctor or physician beforehand to make sure the CBD oil will not inhibit any of those drugs or interact with them negatively. If it does, it likely will not hurt you, but it may reduce the effectiveness of either the CBD or the prescriptions.

One of the most important places to be cautious regarding CBD oil and prescription medications involves any that may be processed by the liver. CBD is thought to interact with the CYP450 system, which is an enzyme in the liver responsible for processing foreign compounds and chemicals that enter the body.

Since this includes many types of prescription medications, CBD can interact negatively with them by causing the liver to process them at a much faster rate than normal and lead to potential disruption of the medication in your system.

Some of the drugs that may be affected by this include:

- Steroids
- Immune modulators
- Antihistamines
- Benzodiazepines
- Calcium channel blockers
- HIV antivirals

Overall, the safety risks and negatives do not outweigh the majority of the benefits regarding CBD oil. Most people who use it for ailments consider it well worth the potential risks, and have reported little to no of the above side effects. This is more of a caution, and a message to stay prepared for any eventuality—nothing is perfect, including CBD!

• Chapter 6 •

Different Forms of CBD and Beginning Use

Most people who have never had any sort of interactions within the cannabis community are often unaware that there are dozens of different strains of cannabis plants. Think of them like trees: there are oaks, pines, willows, and maples. All trees, but all different, and all with their own merit. When it comes to weed smoking, many people like to smoke particular strains to get different effects.

Some are known for 'body highs,' while others stimulate your mind. CBD will not produce the same effects as this marijuana, since they are typically used for their THC content, but there are different strains of marijuana plants and hemp plants specifically geared towards their CBD content and production.

Although legal, CBD products do not undergo the similar federal approval process that medical drugs do, that means it is wide open for errors and the like. CBD products that are being sold at dispensaries possibly have unpredictable concentrations of the compound from patch to batch or even product to product. The quality is inconsistent; therefore, you might go and purchase a product that wonderfully works for you, but when you go back to buy again, you end up finding that the effects are not the same as your first purchase.

There are also well-controlled and well-studied products out in the market by private companies which guarantee consistency and quality CBD products. It is a little expensive than the ones being sold at dispensaries, and harder to get your hands on them, but if you're looking to find CBD products that have consistent compounds, then it is worth the extra bucks.

We briefly touched on a few of the strains earlier, but there are many more out there with varying amounts of CBD in them. The ratios of THC to CBD are extremely important, as you want to get the most out of your chosen strain, and THC will not have the same effects on whatever you are aiming to treat.

To help you get started, I have compiled a list of a few different strains and their CBD/THC percentages, as well as the conditions they are most well-known for helping with:

- **Charlotte's Web:** One of the highest CBD content strains ever, at 20 percent CBD and 0.3 percent THC. This strain is famous for relieving epilepsy symptoms in patients with severe and frequent seizures.
- **ACDC:** Another incredibly high CBD content, at 20 percent CBD and less than 1 percent THC. This strain is known for helping patients with a large variety of conditions, from pain, epilepsy and inflammation to anxiety, PTSD and psychotic symptoms.
- **Harlequin:** This strain clocks in at 15 percent CBD, and around 5 percent THC content. It tends to be more helpful with anxiety, depression and nausea due to its slightly higher THC content.
- **Sour Tsunami:** A slightly lower strain with 11 to 13 percent CBD, but only 0.1 percent THC. Great for helping those who suffer from pains and inflammations, as well as insomnia.

- Cannatonic: This strain never has THC above 6 percent, but its CBD content can range anywhere from 6 to 17 percent. Like many others, this helps with seizures, anxiety, and low blood sugar.
- Avidekel: A man made strain from Israel with about 16 percent CBD and 0 percent THC. This strain is good for treating conditions such as heart diseases, diabetes, inflammations, and arthritis.

Along with these, there are also a couple of rare strains with super high levels of CBD. One of them is called Corazón, and has a CBD percentage of 22.5. This is the single highest level of CBD in a marijuana strain, but it is hard to come by.

This is not a comprehensive list; there are many more strains on the market that help with an ever growing variety of conditions. Some of the strains have a higher THC content so users also get varying degrees of 'high' when they use them, and this can also be known to help with anxieties, depression and body pain. Some strains with a higher THC content for those purposes include:

- Sweet and Sour Widow
- Canna-Tsu
- Pennywise
- Stephen Hawking Kush

Now that you have an introduction to some of the prominent strains in the CBD world, it is time to talk about getting started with dosages and use. Like many other things with CBD, there is no 'one size fits all' option. Dosages can be tricky, as even many physicians are not quite sure yet the amount of CBD to recommend for certain disorders.

This can also be complicated by the many forms that CBD oil comes in. The most common for medical purposes is a dropper, or tincture, that places the CBD directly under your tongue.

While I always recommend consulting a physician before beginning a dosage, there are a couple of ways to attempt to determine it for yourself, especially if your doctor is either unable or unsure how to help. The general rule of thumb is to start on the smaller side, and increase if you feel no effects. You can also use your weight to determine a safe dosage, since the less you weigh, the less you should probably dose.

By this method, many people recommend around 5-10mg (depending on severity of pain) per 25lbs of body weight. Most doses will also vary based on the condition. For example, a person experiencing chronic pains can take a dose as low as 20mg daily and see a noticeable change, where someone with a mental disorder such as schizophrenia can take doses as high as 1000mg per day.

Many CBD products come with a suggested serving size for an average dose. If you are completely new to cannabis as a whole, typically a dose as small as 5mg will be sufficient for the first time to see if you feel any effects. If not, a gradual increase of 5mg per dose until you successfully feel relief is a safe way to test it out.

There is virtually no way to 'overdose' on CBD, so as long as you are careful, consistent and accurate in your dosing there should be no harm. I would not recommend starting with more than 10-20mg for your very first time, unless a higher dose has been recommended by a physician. It is always safer to need more than to need less, after all.

Hopefully this is able to provide you with some of the knowledge you need to choose a strain and a dosage for yourself and get started. There is a lot of contradictory information still out regarding CBD, since so much of the medical community has yet to 'catch up' to the idea of CBD as medicine. However, caution, research and educated attempts go a long way when it comes to trying it, and with such a small risk factor, there is little harm in giving it a shot.

Chapter 7

Physical
Health

One of the most common types of pain people look to treat with CBD oil is body aches, joint problems and arthritis. Chronic pains are the number one reason people regularly visit their physicians, and arthritis is an incredibly common ailment, affecting over 50 million Americans nationwide. It is typically caused by old age and joint wear/inflammation, but it has been known to happen in younger people, as well.

It affects one, many, or even all of the joints in the body by causing swelling, infections, stiffness, and a lack of a range of motion. It is a truly debilitating disease, with no promise of a real treatment or reversal. Once a person begins suffering from it, their only hope is pain management. And unfortunately, many of the traditional treatments for it only have marginal success, with a lot of side effects.

There are two main types of arthritis that CBD is thought to help: rheumatoid arthritis (RA) and osteoarthritis (OA). Rheumatoid arthritis is a disease that causes the body's immune system to attack their own joints, which can make for painful suffering and stiffness. Osteoarthritis is a degenerative problem that goes for cartilage in specific joints.

CBD oil is shown to benefit both of these by working with the CB2 receptors in the body that interact with the immune system, helping the body to reduce inflammation, which reduces pain. Since one of the most oppressive symptoms of arthritis is inflammation, this could be groundbreaking for the future of those who have it.

Not only is CBD oil thought to help relieve the symptoms, it is actually thought to slow the onset of arthritis as well. Many current medications struggle to do this, and also come with some harmful side effects, so the potential for CBD to not only treat but prevent could be life-changing for thousands of people. There have been several studies done on rats and other animals to demonstrate these effects.

One such study took place in 2017. Scientists induced arthritis on a group of male rats, and began monitoring them for pain behavior and blood flow, among other things. They administered the rats with micro doses of CBD, and the results were positive: the CBD effectively blocked the joint pain in the rats, based on their pain behavior.

The CBD also prevented nerve damage in the joints induced with arthritis. This is one example of the future CBD may have in preventing arthritis and helping those who already suffer from it. The potential for CBD to prevent instead of just treat is groundbreaking, as few medicines have ever been thought to truly prevent the onset of this.

Many people who use CBD for arthritis have reported that it works well when combined with other, traditional arthritis medications, and is better still when combined with more consistent exercise and a healthy diet. They also report CBD being more effective when taken orally or topically, combined with injections into the affected joints.

Topically applying CBD, or applying it like a lotion, seems to be one of the most promising methods for this particular ailment, as it allows it to work directly with the inflammation and pain in the joint. It also prevents the CBD from being metabolized by the liver, allowing for more of it to get right into the bloodstream.

Along with arthritic pains, CBD has shown a lot of promise and results in treating other kinds of body pains, such as chronic pains from accidents or diseases and even simple lingering aches. This is where CBD was able to help me; by easing my own chronic pains and allowing me the freedom to take control of my own life and body again.

Chronic pains are recurring, whether for as short as a few weeks or for the rest of your life. They can affect several different areas in the body: the nervous system, muscles, or basic persistent inflammations. CBD is thought to interact with these pains in similar ways it responds to arthritis, by working with the body's pain receptors to shut down some of the signals from the nervous system, and 'block' the pain temporarily.

Since it does this while also helping to reduce the inflammation, it is more than just a typical over the counter pain medication, as it both helps the pain and has the potential to treat the problem all at once.

When attempting to lessen the patient's intake of damaging pain relievers, CBD oil can be a great option when managing the intense pain that arthritis entails. Researchers already acknowledge the fact that CBD plays an important role in alleviating the painful inflammation of arthritis.

Although the effectiveness varies from one individual to the next, it is still worth a try as this is possibly better than your current pain medications.

This is not to say it is a cure, since it's not. It bears repeating that CBD is only a method for pain and possible prevention, but it will not reverse any negative effects you already suffer from. And unfortunately, much of the research has not yet caught up to the results reported by people who use CBD for these conditions.

There has been a shocking amount of positive patient testimony, however, on the use of cannabinoids to treat both those aches and other recurring pains such as headaches and migraines.

One of these positive patient testimonies comes from a man with psoriatic arthritis. He reported quite a bit of pain in the joints and chronic insomnia, along with depression. He started taking just 15mg a day and noticed a world of difference: he could sleep through the night, his pain was manageable, and a drastic improvement in mood. CBD had a trifold effect on his life, raising his overall quality of life and happiness in a very short period of time.

Another patient success story comes from a woman on consistent narcotic use after a bad accident. Narcotics are known for their bad side effects and high rate of addiction, which can cause people to lose their ability to function normally over long periods of time. It can naturally turn those who are on them to look for more natural methods of pain management.

That is what this person did; after years of prescriptions, therapy, and even surgery with no luck, before finally turning to medicinal cannabinoids. She was thrilled with the results: her pain became more tolerable, her moods improved, and she is slowly working on reducing the amount of narcotic medications she takes.

These stories are just two of many like them. Scientists and researchers both agree that there are going to need to be more clinical trials done on these conditions, but that the future is very bright for the use of CBD on those pains. If you are suffering from one of these sorts of pains, CBD may very well be the treatment you are looking for.

If so, then some basic knowledge for getting started involves strains and possible doses. The doses for physical pains and ailments are often much smaller than those used for insomnia or anxiety. This will vary, of course, based on body weight and the type of CBD you are using, but most people report success with doses as low as 5mg to 20mg daily. If you live in a state where marijuana is legal, there have also been positive reports from those who use strains with a slightly higher CBD to THC ratio.

Most strains of CBD have shown to have success in treating body pains, so which one you choose is ultimately up to you and can vary on many factors such as taste, availability, and cost. A couple of the strains we touched on earlier that you may find helpful were ACDC and Sour Tsunami, which have both had some levels of success with pain management.

I wish you the best of luck in managing your chronic pains, and I truly hope that CBD is able to benefit you as it has benefited me. If you have suffered from these pains, then you are all too aware of the toll it can take on your life and the fruitless medical bills that can pile up as a result. Someday soon with any luck, physicians will be able to prescribe CBD as a real treatment and the number of Americans affected can finally begin to drop.

There are all kinds of skin conditions that plague thousands to millions of Americans every year. Some of the worst of these diseases include acne, eczema, hives from allergies, bad reactions and stress, moles, rashes, melanomas, and more.

While these are not usually life-threatening, they can be inconvenient, painful, and damaging to self-esteem and overall happiness and quality of life. While many of these have some form of treatments, from medications to special ointments all the way up to skin graft surgery, many of these options are painful and come with unfortunate and unpleasant side effects.

Chronic problems such as eczema and psoriasis have no real cure, and can only be managed through rigorous treatment. Luckily, both CBD and

THC have been shown to have anti-redness, anti-itch, and help the body fight off overproduction of dendritic and T cells, which both interact with the body's immune system and can cause inflammation.

While there are many skin conditions and CBD has only had clinical trials on a few, there is a lot of hope that its anti-inflammatory benefits may bring relief and healing to those who suffer from these ailments. One is eczema, a painful bumpy and patchy rash that causes dry skin and itchiness. Researchers are not quite sure what it originates from.

However, new evidence and patient testimony's are coming to light that may be positive in regards to CBD as a treatment. Cannabinoids are known for their anti-itch qualities, and CBD promotes the balance of the endocannabinoid system, which helps skin to regulate itself. This will often prevent a lot of the bumps and redness from ever even appearing.

Applying CBD topically to the skin is a popular method of treatment for eczema, and some companies sell lotions and oils specifically for this purpose. It is important before buying, however, to do research on any other ingredients that may be in these products, as some of them could actually do harm to your skin.

Another skin condition CBD may help is psoriasis. Psoriasis is an autoimmune disorder, and it is another incurable condition that causes an overgrowth of skin cells into scaly, painful patches. It can also affect the nails, joints, and scalp. It can eventually lead to arthritis, as well. CBD acts on many of the same effects here as it does for other conditions such as eczema, slowing the rapid growth of skin cells and limiting the buildup. Since psoriasis happens from the inside out, CBD can be used topically for this condition or taken orally.

One skin condition that plagues everybody at some point in their lives, and some for their entire lives, is acne. Acne can range from a few bumps as a teen to incredibly painful cystic acne that can only be cured with extremely harsh treatments.

CBD oil has been used as a topical acne treatment for many people for years, as its anti-inflammatory effects are able to calm the redness and swelling often associated with acne. As with the eczema treatments, there are many products on the internet that advertise as being for CBD treatment as acne, and it is important to be sure if you purchase one that it is a quality, organic treatment and that there are no other harmful chemicals in it, such as alcohols.

While the current scientific evidence regarding CBD as a use for these conditions is limited, there have been a few studies conducted so far. As usual, most of these have been done on mice or rats, but there have been a couple of reasonably successful ones on humans. One such study looked to test the relationship between cannabinoids and the immune system by testing how it affected the itching in patients with uremic pruritus, a condition caused by kidney problems.

They applied the CBD topically with a cream 2 times a day for 3 weeks. They were met with varying results; in 8 of the 21 patients, the problem completely disappeared, but others only had more limited results or success. This of course does not discount the success found in the 8 patients, as even a 40 percent success rate is too high to be ignored for long.

This sums up much of the trials that have been done so far on CBD and skin conditions. Many people who try it as an herbal remedy have been very pleased with it, but many more clinical studies will need to be done before conclusive results can be confirmed.

Autoimmune diseases and disorders are another branch of medicine people are hoping to treat with CBD oil. There are dozens of diseases and conditions that are caused by the immune system turning on itself and attacking the body, such as lupus, celiac disease, Chron's disease, fibromyalgia, and endometriosis, to name just a few.

While much of these diseases are still not quite understood by researchers, there are a few basic things about autoimmune diseases we do know: they can affect any part of the body, from the GI tract, to the joints, to skin (as we just covered); they can last only a short time, or be recurring throughout a person's entire life; they are very difficult to treat, since the problem is the person's own body; and they seem to be caused by a number of things, but in layman's terms something within the body recognizes something else as foreign and attacks it. This can be a response to poor diet, overactive hormones, or certain types of viruses.

Here, we will take a look at Chron's disease. Chron's is an inflammatory disease that affects the gastrointestinal tract, particularly the bowels. In the worst cases it can be debilitating, and it often causes excruciating pain in patients. It's often genetic, and there is no cure. The best one can hope for at this point is a rigid schedule of prescription medications to manage the symptoms and pain.

CBD may able to change that, however. The same anti-inflammatory effects that make CBD so effective on skin conditions are able to come into play here, reducing the inflammation and swelling within the GI tract to allow relief. CBD has also been demonstrated to relieve pain and allow for better sleep in these patients, also curbing the nausea and diarrhea that are common symptoms of Chron's.

There has been more conclusive research done on medical marijuana and Chron's, and it has even been approved in 22 states to treat the disease, so CBD may soon follow as an effective treatment.

There are many stories of success on the Internet involving CBD and Chron's. One comes from a teen diagnosed in 2011. For several years, he suffered, enduring terrible debilitating pains, slowed growth, and causing him to lose both weight and quality of life. His family turned to CBD oil as a last result, and like many others they were stunned by the improvement. Within a year he had gained weight back, was pain free and his inflammation and ulcers had all but disappeared.

Chron's is just one of many; there are many other autoimmune diseases that people have reported being calmed by regular use of CBD oil, like endometriosis and lupus. Unfortunately, there is virtually no scientific evidence yet to back it up, so personal testimonies are the most important factors to consider, and the evidence from other diseases CBD has helped.

There are several decent studies done on medical marijuana to treat many of these diseases, but CBD oil itself is still a relatively new product and must 'catch up' to the rest of the industry. However, if medical marijuana is able to help, then that bodes well for the future of CBD oil, too.

The most important thing to be aware of before attempting CBD oil relief for an autoimmune disease is to consider any other medications you may be taking regularly, even if they are just over the counter pain medications. Since many people with these conditions can take a wide variety of meds to help with them, it is more important than ever to discuss it with your physician beforehand.

Cancer

Cancer comes in many forms and varies in the complications that they entail: breast, lung, carcinomas, leukemic, pancreatic, lymphomas, and many more. It can be benign or malignant. There are over 100 different types of cancer, some of which are mild and easy to treat, and some of which can turn deadly within weeks. Everybody knows someone whose lives have been impacted by some form of this disease.

Cancer is characterized by the overgrowth of cells. Typically, old cells stop dying and new ones begin dividing at a rapid rate, causing masses of cells called tumors. Benign tumors can often be removed and will not grow back, but a malignant tumor sometimes will, and can spread to other parts of the body.

They can become quite large, impacting organs and halting normal functions. Tumors can, in a sense, reprogram the body to provide them with what they need to continue growing. Because tumors are made up of a person's own cells and tissue, they are extremely hard to kill.

Cancer can be caused by many things. Genetics, exposure to chemicals, excessive UV rays (the sun), obesity, smoking, and gene mutations, to name just a few. The most common treatment options include radiation, surgery, and chemotherapy. Unfortunately, depending on the severity of the cancer, these treatments often only have moderate levels of success, especially if the cancer spread before it was detected.

People have searched for alternative treatments to cancer for decades. Almost all of them are unproven, such as aromatherapy, strange diets, magnetic therapy, and an unending range of holistic medicines and brews promoted by strangers on the internet. There is virtually no science to back most of these up, and often people turn to these out of sheer desperation.

CBD and medical marijuana, however, may provide an additional cancer treatment that could be backed by science. It is not likely that either of these things will be able to fight cancer entirely on their own, but when combined with traditional cancer treatments, people have found varying levels of success.

Some studies have shown that marijuana can lessen the nausea and vomiting associated with chemotherapy, as well as increasing appetite, which is typically affected due to the radiation. One drug, Dronabinol, is a capsule containing THC that has been approved for use in chemotherapy patients to reduce their nausea during treatment.

Of course, CBD is a different compound, used for slightly different things. In cancer patients, it has benefits for aiding with nausea relief and pain management. Researchers are hopeful, however, that it has potential to actually inhibit tumor growth, as well. One study done back in 2006 looked at five different compounds (cannabidiol, cannabigerol, cannabichromene, cannabidiol acid and THC acid) to test which one had the strongest breast tumor growth inhibitors.

Of the five, cannabidiol (CBD) tested the strongest, believed to be because of interaction with CB2 receptors. The researchers agreed that, while more testing is going to be needed on CBD oil and tumor growth, it should be done.

Since that year, there has been some more examination into the abilities of CBD against cancer. Another trial used mice to examine CBD against leukemia and lymphoblasts. The researchers found that the cannabidiol acting on CB2 receptors may target irregular cell growth and help the immune system fight off and kill the malignant cells.

This could, with more studies, possibly mean that CBD can help the body prevent tumor growth altogether. Once the tumors have grown, CBD does not appear to be able to get rid of them, but the potential for slowing growth and calming the side effects could mean volumes for cancer patients.

Many people are already self-medicating with CBD during their cancerous stages. Although science has yet to back it up, some are even reporting that their supposedly terminal tumors have yet to take their lives solely because of CBD treatments. This is likely due to a variety of factors, and not just CBD, but the overwhelming amount of success stories is still a positive development for those looking for alternative cancer treatments.

Some people have had success with high THC strains of medical marijuana, but some prefer CBD for its anti-psychoactive effects, especially for adolescents. Many turn to it as a last resort, and are surprised by how much it ends up helping. Although the doses people were administering for anti-cancer regimens were much higher than other ailments, sometimes up to a gram a day, but any potential side effects seem to be considered well worth it for the benefits.

The biggest consideration with CBD and cancer seems to be taking consistent daily doses over weeks or months, so that the CBD can continue to work with CB1 and CB2 receptors to inhibit the cell growth and kill the metastasized cells.

One woman from the UK reported that she had terminal cancer in two places on her body: her collar bone, and her anal canal. The doctors told her she had a year, if not months, to live, but she was hesitant to do radiation therapy due to the burns. She turned to CBD oil, ingesting it and applying it topically, and one year later returned to the doctor to incredible news—her cancer was completely gone.

Another Unites States based 2 year old boy was diagnosed with leukemia, and given a very slim chance of survival. Chemotherapy caused him intense pain, among other unpleasant and debilitating side effects, and his parents turned to CBD oil to try and help him survive more comfortably. Within weeks, they noticed a difference, and now the boy is 5 years old and still in remission with no chemotherapy whatsoever.

These are just two of hundreds of success stories out there. Like dozens of other illnesses and problems, CBD is rising to the surface as an incredible new herbal treatment with real potential and significantly fewer side effects than traditional cancer treatments. This is one of the bonuses for many people, as chemotherapy and radiation do sometimes eliminate the cancer, but the side effects from them can linger for the rest of your life.

Strains that have been reported to be beneficial to cancer victims are ACDC and Harlequin, and if you don't mind a higher THC content, people have reported success with marijuana strains like Northern Lights and Skywalker OG. Keep in mind, however, that these are often used to treat the side effects of cancer and cancer treatments, like nausea, pain, and appetite loss, instead of the cancer itself. For use with the side effects, people have reported success with dosages as low as 2.5mg per day.

If you are looking to completely replace traditional cancer treatments with CBD oil, then your dose is going to vary widely based on body weight, type of cancer, severity of cancer, and any treatments or medications you may be using or have used in the past. This is one of the cases where it is more important than ever to be thorough, since cancer is such a serious illness.

That being said, as far as last ditch efforts go, it may be time for the medical community to stop considering CBD as one, and to start seeing it as a real treatment with a viable place in the cancer community.

Gastrointestinal Problems

Gastrointestinal diseases can cover a wide range of disorders. The human digestive tract is surprisingly large, and covers intestines from the mouth and throat down through the stomach, large and small intestines, colon, and more. A few of the things impacted by the GI tracts we are going to take a look at here include appetite, nausea, irritable bowel problems, and even how appetite affects eating disorders, although those can be classified as mental illnesses as well.

Appetite loss is a common side effect of many other diseases, from ones as simple and treatable as colds or the flu to the more serious problems associated with cancer or Chron's disease. Long term appetite loss is almost always a result of something larger, like pregnancy or the aforementioned diseases, and it can even be a side effect of mental conditions such as depression or anxiety, or drug abuse.

It can also be a problem all on its own, and loss of the ability to properly eat affects every other function within the human body. CBD has been reported by many to help with appetite loss, and stimulates it in patients who may be suffering with this problem. This is especially crucial in people with eating disorders like anorexia or bulimia, who sometimes go for so long without eating that feeling normal hunger and the desire for food becomes difficult.

So, while appetite loss can happen for a range of reasons, appetite stimulation is incredibly important in those who have lost it. Unhealthy weight loss tends to follow, and extreme and sudden weight loss can come with all sorts of other medical complications, and can even turn deadly if it goes too far.

Traditional treatments for this are typically prescription medications, which come with their own side effects and problems, and do not always help the problem at hand. THC is typically known as the cannabis product that stimulates hunger, since it is believed to bind to CB1 receptors and create 'the munchies.' CBD does not do this, but researchers believe it stimulates hunger in other ways: by reducing inflammation, stress, and other factors in the body that decrease appetite. By helping to eliminate those issues, people are more comfortable eating.

This is particularly important in those with eating disorders. Research has shown that those with anorexia have underperforming endocannabinoid systems, and CBD is able to stimulate this. It will not get rid of the problem, but by helping provide homeostasis and calming other issues related to eating disorders such as anxiety, people are more likely to be able to stimulate hunger and eat with less anxiety.

There have been no clinical studies on this yet, but a treatment other than prescription medications and therapy may be extremely beneficial to those with this problem.

Nausea, on the other hand, does have some scientific backing behind CBD as a treatment. Researchers believe CBD has anti-emetic effects, which literally means it prevents vomiting. The only other treatments for nausea are medications, whether over the counter or prescription, but those often come with side effects such as drowsiness, diarrhea or headaches. Nausea can, like appetite loss, be caused by a variety of factors, including migraines, motion sickness, pain, as a side effect of other diseases or medications, and pregnancy.

There have been many more studies done on THC and nausea than CBD, but researchers are looking into CBD as a treatment. One study was done on rats, to see if CBD was able to prevent nausea reactions. Since rats can't vomit, they conditioned the rats to gape their mouth and retch in the presence of typical nausea-inducing things. They found that both THC and CBD were effective in preventing these gape responses, and suspect this may be due to CBDs interaction with CB1 receptors and by triggering 5-HT1A.

Those who take CBD for appetite problems or nausea reduction typically ingest it with sprays, by vaping or with tinctures (dropper placed under the tongue). This is one place where edibles are not typically the most effective, especially since they take so long to kick in. The average dose varies, but for more short term problems such as these, erring on the side of smaller doses is a good idea. If a little does not help, you can always take more, but since one of the more commonly reported side effects of CBD can be nausea it is best to be careful.

Irritable bowel syndrome (sometimes referred to as colitis) is another incurable disorder characterized by painful cramping, bloating, diarrhea, and constipation. It is chronic, and can be lifelong. While doctors are not quite sure what causes it in particular patients, they do know that it happens when abnormal muscle contractions or problems in the nervous system, and can cause inflammations and infections in the GI system. It can easily be triggered by stress or certain types of foods, and greatly lowers overall quality of life.

While there is not a ton of evidence out yet supporting CBD as a treatment for this condition, there have been a few studies on THC and IBS, and researchers are hopeful CBD will be able to reduce the inflammation and muscle spasms common in this disorder. The endocannabinoid system interacts heavily with the digestive system, and helps the body regulate these functions.

One study in 2011 tested the ability of cannabidiol to treat mice with ulcerative colitis, a very similar condition to IBS. They found that CBD led to a decrease in the inflammation and macrophages, which are commonly found at the site of infections. Another study done on patients with ulcerative colitis tested CBD and found that the treatments were effectively able to reduce intestinal inflammation and bring relief.

Along with these studies are a good amount of patient testimonies verifying the results of this product. One reported a lifetime of chronic IBS, accompanied by cramping, vomiting, and debilitating pain. Medications were unable to bring true relief, so finally they turned to CBD oil, taking as little as 5mg per day with an additional vaporizer. The results were profound: the attacks subsided to infrequently, the pain was barely noticeable if present at all, and years of pain finally came to an end.

CBD oils potential to help muscle spasms and inflammation could be life changing for people with gastrointestinal problems. As with the nausea and vomiting, it seems to work best for these conditions with tinctures and vaporizers, but if you want longer term results you can try edibles as well.

Since CBD treatment for the conditions covered in this chapter tend to go along with other medications (i.e. if you are nauseous s due to another condition), be sure that the CBD will not interact with any medications. This is especially important if the nausea is related to larger problems, such as cancer.

As more people report on the effectiveness of CBD to treat these conditions, the research community also pushes for more clinical trials. With any luck, these will continue to illuminate what we already suspect: that CBD is a more than viable treatment for GI problems, and should be a valid part of the medical community.

Neurodegenerative Diseases

Some of the most inhibitive diseases known to man are neurodegenerative diseases, such as Parkinson's, Huntington's, and Multiple Sclerosis, to name just a few. They are completely incurable, and few treatments are able to help the symptoms. They can affect movement, like Parkinson's, or mental cognition, like dementia.

Parkinson's disease takes place within the central nervous system, and almost entirely affects adults and the elderly, although cases have been reported in people as low as their teens. Once someone has it, it is chronic and lifelong, with the only hope to slow the symptom progression as long as possible. Some of the symptoms of Parkinson's are tremors, stiffness in the muscles, slurred speech, cognitive dysfunction, and slow movement. Researchers are not quite sure what causes it, but genetics and environmental factors may play a role.

Parkinson's affects the neurons in the substantia nigra in the brain, which is an area that produces the neurotransmitter dopamine. It can cause dopamine to be at much lower than normal levels, or to be completely absent in more severe cases. This is a problem because, among other things, dopamine helps the body to move normally. And like many other conditions CBD helps to treat, the endocannabinoid system plays a role in Parkinson's, although researchers are just now beginning to understand it.

So, how can CBD help with this? Traditional medicines and treatments only treat the symptoms at best, with a range of unpleasant side effects, but CBD may be able to do a little more. One study conducted in 2014 aimed to test the abilities of medical marijuana on Parkinson's symptoms such as tremors. 22 patients were tested for their pain levels and motor skills before and after the administering of the marijuana.

The results and reports from the patients demonstrated decreased pain, better ability to sleep, and significant lowering of tremors. While this particular test was on marijuana and not CBD, it still positively demonstrates the potential for such treatments.

The current research points towards CBD aiding in dopamine production, which helps the body with regulation motor functions. One study tested this on 21 people with PD by giving them either a placebo, 75mg of CBD, or 300mg of CBD. During this time, the researchers monitored their motor functions, quality of life, and neuro-activity in the brain.

The findings were slightly inconclusive; there was no drastic difference, but those who received the higher 300mg dose of CBD showed an improvement in quality of life over those who had received the placebo. Overall, the researchers agreed this could be beneficial in the future, but that more studies need to be done first.

Between the studies involving medical marijuana, the suspected role CBD plays in the endocannabinoid system and with dopamine receptors, and a surprising amount of patient testimony, there is certainly enough evidence to back up giving CBD a shot for Parkinson's treatments. The side effects from CBD are far lesser than side effects from traditional Parkinson's medications, and the hope for relief from PD symptoms shouldn't be ignored.

Huntington's disease, which is much rarer than PD, is another chronic, progressively worsening disease that attacks neurons in the brain. This one is genetic, passed down entirely through inheritance. It is similar to Parkinson's in many ways, typically not setting in until later in life and with characteristic difficulty moving, muscle problems, involuntary movement, and cognitive dysfunction. Since it makes day to day tasks so difficult, it can greatly decrease overall quality of life, and often comes with mental health problems as a side effect of that.

Huntington's targets several different areas in the brain, including the substantia nigra, cerebral cortex, hippocampus, and hypothalamus, to name a few. The most prominent area of the brain targeted by HD, however, is the basil ganglia, an area dedicated to motor control and functions. The nerve death caused there is irreversible and can lead to complete lack of motor control by the end stages of the disease. Even in today's modern world, there are very few treatments that provide any kind of relief or assistance to those with HD, even just to curb the symptoms.

One study was done by GW Pharmaceuticals to test equal amounts of THC and CBD together on patients with HD. The results were underwhelming, but not necessarily bad—the patients showed no ill effects due to the cannabinoids, but they also showed little change in their movement or cognitive functions. This did not deter the researchers, however, who said that this only drives the fuel for more studies to be done. The antioxidant effects of CBD are very promising as a potential treatment for HD.

One last neurodegenerative disease to take a look at is Multiple Sclerosis. MS can be categorized as both an autoimmune disorder and a neurodegenerative disorder, since it is caused by the immune system attacking the protective covering over nerves and destroying it. This can cause damage to nerves all over the central nervous system of the brain and spinal cord.

Like other neurodegenerative diseases, it is progressive and incurable, and can only be treated for the symptoms once it is caught. It causes cognitive problems, vision problems, pain, muscle spasms, and weakness, and even seizures, hearing loss, and other complications. MS is a chronic condition that can last anywhere from years to being lifelong. It also varies widely in severity, with some people having manageable, treatable symptoms and others having severe chronic issues their entire lives.

New research is coming out that CBD may be able to help with MS. It is believed to do so by diminishing pain, muscle problems, and aiding in sleep, as well as slowing the progression of nerve damage and helping overall motor functions. CBD oils ability to calm muscle spasms can greatly improve the day to day functions and lives of those with MS, since these spasms can cause problems in many ordinary and basic aspects of life.

An article published in 2018 discussed the potential for CBD benefits for MS, citing the anti-inflammatory and antioxidant effects of cannabinoids. Researchers are hopeful that it can also benefit cognitive brain function that gets damaged by MS, aiding in common symptoms like anxiety and memory problems. The equal 1:1 ratio of THC and CBD seems especially promising in neurological disorders as a whole.

While there is a significant amount of studying and clinical trials left to be done on neurodegenerative diseases, many people with these conditions have reported levels of success with CBD treatments. One of the biggest factors across these patient testimonies has been consistent dosing. Since MS does not typically go away, it is important to stay stringent and maintain the CBD levels to get the desired results. This is worth remembering for the use of CBD with any neurological disease.

CBD has been administered in a variety of ways and been effective, from tinctures and rubbing it into the skin as well as edibles. The average dose remains fairly low, as well, starting at around 20-30mg per day to get baseline results.

Although neurodegenerative diseases are one of the areas with the least clinical trials done on CBD, the amount of hope researchers have as this for a future treatment speaks well for patients. Unlike many other conditions, which have decent levels of success with more traditional medications, neurological problems are still extremely difficult to effectively treat, making the potential for CBD as an effective solution that much greater.

Alzheimer's

While Alzheimer's falls into the same category of diseases as other neurological disorders, its effects are nearly entirely cognitive instead of physical. It is extremely common, affecting more than 4 million Americans every year. It is almost always found in older people. In other developed countries and in the United States, Alzheimer's disease is one of the primary causes of dementia and there is no cure for it or method to slow down its progression at all, although there are some treatments that can ease the effects of the symptoms.

Alzheimer's is a progressive disease that begins in the hippocampus, the part of the brain that controls memory. Scientists are not sure what causes it, and suspect it is a combination of factors including genetics, environment, and overall health. The brain damage can begin years before symptoms start to show up, making it extremely hard to effectively treat or prevent, since there is no reversal of the damage.

This takes place in the brain by an excessive, irregular buildup of proteins that turn into plaques on the nerve cells. This makes the nerves start to break down and collapse, shrinking and spreading throughout the entire brain. It can cause dementia, inability to care for one's self, hallucinations, and difficulty moving or talking properly. It can take years to become fatal, but destroys thought processes, leaving the patient with very little trace of who they once were and virtually no good quality of life.

There are a few different stages that Alzheimer's can be caught in: mild, moderate, and severe. Once it is diagnosed, doctors have to act quickly to have any hope of maintaining healthy cognitive functions for as long as possible. This is done with prescription medications, exercise and diet, and daily routines to help the patient establish habits. While these are great for trying to improve the overall health and well-being of the patient, they are still extremely limited and the effects typically only last a few years at best.

Any disease with such low, if not nonexistent, rates of repair can cause people to look for other treatments to help. Luckily, they may have found one in CBD oil. While it is unlikely that THC or CBD can prevent the onset of Alzheimer's, there is some belief that it may be able to benefit the brain by helping to remove the plaque buildup that damages the nerves.

It helps in many of the same ways it helps the body with other neurodegenerative diseases: with its anti-inflammatory and antioxidant effects, preventing neuron breakdown, and boosting the endocannabinoid system. It also targets a range of other neurotransmitters, such as glutamate receptors and 5-HT1A.

There have not been any documented clinical trials yet on CBD oil and human Alzheimer's, but a few studies have been conducted on animals, namely rats. A group of adult male rats was induced with Alzheimer's, and then given 10mg of CBD oil a day for 15 days. The researchers found that CBD oils anti-inflammatory effects were able to help restore and aid the brain in neuron protection.

Another similar study, also done on rats induced with Alzheimer's, injected them with 20mg of CBD oil once daily for a week, and then dropped the treatments back to 3 times a week for another two weeks. Interestingly, they found that the CBD treated rats had some of their cognitive damage reversed, while the control rats (those who did not receive the CBD) showed no change.

There have been several other studies done on mice and rats to study the effects of CBD on Alzheimer's related neuron damage, with varying ranges of success, but the important thing to note is that they all did in fact have a level of success. It has also been demonstrated that equal parts THC and CBD may be even more effective against neurodegenerative diseases, since the THC is able to combine with the CBD and act on slightly different systems.

Researchers believe that this only further drives the need for proper clinical trials, since no other treatments have been found to be truly effective against Alzheimer's and the potential for one to actually slow down its progression could be life changing for millions of people worldwide.

Along with these preclinical trials are testimonies from patients pledging to the success of CBD oil, and medical marijuana/THC as well. Many people have tried it out on their loved ones, to see if it could bring any sort of cognitive recognition or resemblance of normal function back. One man began giving his mother THC-infused brownies shortly after her diagnosis of Alzheimer's, and reported that in six months her condition had not worsened in the slightest.

Another shockingly positive success story comes from someone with a mother in their 90s, who had been diagnosed with dementia, Alzheimer's, and had suffered a stroke at 85. She was not able to talk or move her limbs with any comfort. They began giving her CBD both orally and topically, and her condition gradually improved so that she is not only able to move her arms and legs more, but can also speak clearly on occasion.

Along with these two stories are an incredible amount of videos out there, physically demonstrating the effects CBD has on Alzheimer's patients. In many of them you can see the change before and after the CBD is administered daily for even as little as a week at a time. Nearly catatonic patients become able to speak progressively more clearly as the treatments go on, they are more aware of their surroundings, and they can move more freely.

The average dosing for Alzheimer's treatment is much higher than the doses for other conditions. The recommended doses get higher based on the severity of the condition, but even for those who have early stages of the disease many people recommend starting at around 4mg of CBD oil per pound of body weight daily. For severe cases, this can be increased gradually per day.

The recommended strains for treatment of Alzheimer's are typically hybrid strains, which means they have equally higher ratios of THC and CBD. In states where marijuana and medical marijuana are not legal yet, though, or if you simply want to avoid the psychoactive effects (the 'high') then some CBD strains recommended are ACDC, The OX, and Harlequin. These strains are known for their slightly higher THC content, but are still available in most states in CBD oil form, making them a more universal treatment for Alzheimer's.

If you or a loved one are looking to treat Alzheimer's with cannabis products, the general consensus among many seems to be to give it a go. Since there are literally no other treatments that provide true long term benefits with the disease, and those all come with unpleasant side effects, the only way to go is up.

Even if CBD is not able to provide the answer, and it may not be as everyone varies, the lack of side effects make it a viable option to at least try. With any luck, it will at the very least be able to provide the patient with more motor function and cognitive ability then they may have had previously, or prolong the function they have if they are still in the early stages of Alzheimer's.

Alzheimer's is a truly terrible ailment that causes suffering not only to the patient, but to their loved ones as they watch them physically and mentally deteriorate over the years. Hopefully, CBD oil and cannabinoids will continue to be pushed through and tested as a valid treatment, so that the new generations will have a little less to worry about as they get older.

COPD

Chronic Obstructive Pulmonary Disease, or COPD, is a chronic, incurable disease that affects several million Americans across the country, and is listed as the third leading cause of death annually. It causes inflammation in the lungs that block airflow, and it can be an effect of other diseases such as bronchitis or emphysema. It is typically caused by smoking or, in some cases, too much inhalation of secondhand smoke. It can also be a result of factors like working in a dusty environment for too long, genetic predisposition, or living in areas with high air pollution.

Symptoms of COPD generally include coughing, mucus buildup, inability to draw full breaths, swelling, and respiratory infections. It is very treatable, unlike many of the other conditions covered within this book, but once a person has it there is little chance of it ever healing or going away.

While treatable, those treatments usually consist of improved self-health care, inhalers, steroids and antibiotics, oxygen therapy (such as using an oxygen mask at night) and surgery in extreme cases. Untreated COPD can lead to many other complications, though, such as pneumonia, heart attacks, or cancer, as well as mental illnesses such as depression.

CBD oil may be able to benefit those with COPD by reducing inflammation within the lungs. It has been demonstrated many times to be effective at lowering inflammation in all parts of the body, from the joints and skin to inner organs. It does this by activating the body's CB1 and CB2 receptors in the endocannabinoid, influencing proper homeostasis and thereby improving overall lung functions.

It also helps the body rid itself of excessive T cells and dendritic cells, which flock to areas with inflammation and infection. By doing this, the airways are allowed more room to expand and let airflow through.

There are some clinical trials currently underway to test CBD on COPD, but no results have as of yet been posted. However, one study back in 2011 did a double-blind, placebo based trial to test the effectiveness of CBD oil on breathlessness in those with and without COPD. Five healthy subjects and four with COPD received either a placebo or 10mg of CBD over a two day period.

They were then measured for breathlessness, mood, and ventilation before, during, and after the trial. The results showed that there was not much of a change, but that the patients who received the CBD had less 'air hunger,' or what could be described as a suffering from lack of proper airflow.

While these results are not particularly impressive or groundbreaking, they do demonstrate the need for many more studies and tests to be done. It was also a very small, short term trial, which may have impacted its potential. One interesting thing to note is that while CBD may be able to assist in inhibiting the inflammation, this condition can actually be worsened by smoking marijuana (with THC in it) on a regular basis.

The crucial aspect here seems to be how the product is ingested, and not the chemical itself. This can change and depend on who you ask, however, as some people have reported moderate levels of relief by smoking marijuana, claiming it helps to relax the lung muscles and allow for easier breathing.

The trick here seems to be to stay cautious with ingestion, especially if your preferred method is vaporizing CBD. Until more clinical trials can be done on the actual interaction with CBD and COPD, it is best to steer completely clear of this method. Instead, choose one of the other ways to ingest CBD oil: through edibles, tinctures (dropper under the tongue), topically applying either the oil or an infused cream/lotion, or even an inhaler.

Depending on your state, treating the COPD may become tricky. No states in the US have yet to approve CBD oil as a valid treatment for COPD, and if you are still in one of the four with murky laws regarding CBD, this may be worth investigating before attempting it.

If you would like to try CBD oil to help with your COPD or other inflammatory airway problems, first make sure that it will not inhibit any other treatments you may be using, such as inhalers or steroids. CBD has been shown before to interact with the CYP450 system, an enzyme in the liver responsible for metabolizing foreign compounds, many of which include prescription medications and other drugs.

CBD can make this enzyme process faster, which can lead to higher levels than normal of other drugs in your system, and cause accidental overdoses (this is not to say fatal overdoses, but still higher than normal and could be unhealthy). Steroids are processed by this same enzyme, so it is crucial to consult your physician before beginning a CBD treatment for COPD.

If you have talked to your doctor and received the go-ahead to try CBD oil, the average dosing for treating COPD symptoms seem to start as low as 50mg a few times a week, with the potential for increase if needed. Since COPD tends to be chronic, many recommend attempting it over the course of a few weeks to start, and if you see no visible improvements in that time it may not be the choice for you. Hopefully, though, that will not be the case, and CBD will be able to benefit your lung issues as well as it has benefited others.

Epilepsy and Seizures

Many of the most groundbreaking studies and research done on CBD oil have involved epilepsy and seizures. It is the most famous disease or ailment that is helped by CBD, and has been demonstrated numerous times to almost completely stop seizures in dozens of people over several clinical trials. There have even been specified laws regarding CBD based entirely on the possession of CBD for the use of treating epilepsy, such as "Carly's Law" in Alabama, which is the only law in the state that allows for the possession of medical CBD oil.

Epilepsy, or seizure disorder, is a neurological problem that affects over 200,000 people every year. It can be inherited, or a result of other health problems such as strokes, head injury, and other medical complications. There are a few kinds of epilepsy, and it knows no age. Someone who has epilepsy usually has to live with it for life, although there are some individuals who suffer for only a short amount of time, and the seizures just go away.

Anybody can have a seizure, yet it does not mean that he or she already has epilepsy. If a person had more than just one seizure, and the doctors are convinced that it will be reoccurring, then that is the only time a person is diagnosed. While it does not usually affect the patient between seizures, people can have anywhere from a couple a year to up to a hundred a day. They greatly affect quality of life, as the most severe cases often can't lead normal, everyday lives and activities.

Most epilepsy is a chronic and lifelong condition that never truly goes away and can only be treated. Some people have found relative success and comfort from traditional medicines, but some are completely not helped by those or are affected negatively by the side effects. These are often the people who benefit from CBD oil treatments.

Epilepsy happens when groups of neurons suddenly begin firing in the brain at times they shouldn't. CBD interacts with this by regulating the rate of neural firing and preventing it altogether, effectively 'quieting' the brains neural action. There are two main types of epileptic seizures CBD has been shown to help with: Lennox-Gastaut syndrome, and Dravet syndrome.

Lennox-Gastaut is characterized by frequent seizures that begin in childhood, and has some sort of moderate to severe mental disabilities. Dravet syndrome typically begins in infancy, with seizures onset by fevers or being hot.

Charlotte Figi is one of the most famous cases of children who have benefited from CBD oil. She suffers from Dravet syndrome, which onset before she was a year old. Her seizures would happen multiple times daily and would sometimes last as long as four hours.

She was on heavy prescription medications, which side effects combined with the seizures began to take a noticeable toll both on her mental health and her quality of life. Her condition worsened, to the point she was having 300 seizures a week. Her parents were all but ready to say their last goodbyes and let her go. She was five years old at the time.

At the time, both CBD and medical marijuana were very tough to come by. After a lot of digging, they were able to find some CBD oil and test it on Charlotte, and they were astonished at the results: the seizures stopped. With regular administration, she had no seizures for an entire week. The Stanley Brothers, who Charlotte's parents had gotten the CBD from, even ended up naming the strain of marijuana after Charlotte. This is the origin of the Charlotte's Web strain.

Today, Charlotte is living an almost completely normal life. She still gets two doses of CBD a day, and only has seizures two or three times a month. Her story has spread across the nation, and has helped countless other children with similar conditions to improve.

This is one of the most emotional and impactful stories demonstrating the effects that CBD can have on a person's life. It is entirely likely Charlotte may never have recovered had her parents not discovered CBD and began administering it to her, and she would have never had a shot at being a normal child.

Along with the success stories such as Charlotte's, many of the major case studies done on CBD have had to do with epilepsy. One was the first study done on humans to test CBD oil as a medical treatment in 1980, which is discussed in more depth in Chapter 22. Another was conducted in 2017 in Europe.

Researchers gathered 120 adolescents with Dravet syndrome, and divided them into two groups, one which would receive CBD oil treatments and one which would receive a placebo. The test lasted longer than normal ones, at 3 and ½ months. By the end, the results showed that those who had received the CBD oil had almost half as many seizures as before, while the placebo group showed little change.

One noteworthy effect of this study was more reported side effects, but those being tested were still on their old seizure medications, so there is some speculation that this may have interacted negatively with the CBD to create those effects.

Regardless, the drop in seizures is certainly positive, and continues to perpetrate the evidence for CBD as a legitimate drug against seizures. In 2018, the

FDA approved the first CBD based drug, Epidiolex, designated to treat both Dravet and Lennox-Gastaut syndrome. This is a huge step forward for CBD, and for those who suffer from epilepsy. It does come with side effects, although not as many as prescription drugs, some of which are drowsiness, appetite increase or decrease, diarrhea, insomnia, and some mild liver damage.

Many people still use regular CBD oil instead of Epidiolex for their seizures, however. Some of the most popular strains for this treatment are, of course, Charlotte's Web, Avidekel, and Cannatonic. There have also been reports that doses as low as 10mg once or twice a day can still have a significant effect on seizures.

With a condition like epilepsy, it is not only a good idea to discuss it with your physician beforehand, it is almost essential. With the recent FDA approval of a CBD based drug, at the very least you can be sure that trying CBD will not negatively interact with any current prescription medications you may be taking, but depending on your state you may also be able to be prescribed CBD. This takes a lot of the pressure out of trying to find a good product, since you will be able to get it through stricter sources that have checked into the creation of the product.

If epilepsy is the condition you are looking to treat, you're in luck—the cannabis community is an excellent resource to help you on this journey, and medical marijuana is a viable option as well if CBD doesn't quite fit your needs. Stories of success regarding seizures only grow every year, and hopefully yours or your loved ones will be one of them!

Heart Diseases

There are several different types of cardiovascular dysfunctions, or heart diseases. These can include heart attacks (also called cardiac arrest), heart failure, arrhythmia, coronary artery disease, high blood pressure, strokes, and many more. There are too many specific diseases to full list off them all and their symptoms, but overall heart health is something millions of Americans worry about on an annual basis.

The heart is absolutely vital to all of the body's functions, since without it there would be no way to get oxygen to vital organs, cells, and even the brain. When one thing goes wrong with the heart, it can start to go wrong everywhere else, too.

Heart diseases can be caused by a variety of things. Stress, drug abuse, age, birth defects, smoking, and even as a result of some prescription medications, to name just a few. It is not likely that something will go wrong with your heart without a cause, whether it be genetic or otherwise. Many of the common symptoms in those affected by heart disease include pain in the chest, legs, and arms; irregular heartbeats; shortness of breath; fatigue; dizziness; and even fevers.

Many heart problems can be fatal, whether it be very quickly like heart attacks or over a period of time, like high blood pressure. The most important treatment is to take care of your body and diet as well as possible, but unfortunately other factors can come into play even when doing that. The most common treatments for heart conditions are diet changes, prescription medications, and for more extreme cases, surgeries, pacemakers, and even heart transplants, although the latter is extremely hard to come by.

None of these is ideal to the patient, since prescription medications can cause damage to other parts of the body and the stress of pacemakers and surgery can be fatal when things go wrong as well.

However, medical marijuana and CBD may be able to change the face of the heart health industry. Doctors and researchers are extremely hopeful that CBD will be able to benefit many areas impacted by negative heart health, such as inflammation, poor sleep, and to aid in improving circulation. There has been a rising amount of research done in the last few years to show the effects of both THC and CBD on heart health.

One such study took place in 2017. A group of researchers gathered 9 healthy males and gave them either a placebo or a 600mg dose of CBD oil and monitored their blood pressure and mental stress. Off of just one dose, they found that those who had received the CBD had lower resting blood pressure rates and stress, but slightly higher heart rates.

Another trial conducted in 2010 tested CBD treatments on rats with induced coronary artery occlusion, which means the rats had certain arteries essentially blocked off to mimic heart conditions. This caused arrhythmias, dead cells, and mast cell problems in the rats.

They found that the rats who had received the micro dosing of CBD had lower rates of arrhythmia and fewer of the dead cells, also called infarcts, although there was very little change between the two groups in mass cells. The researchers believe that this may be because of CBDs influence on CB1 receptors. These two studies conclusively demonstrate that CBD may in fact have a future in heart health.

More studies certainly need to be done, but the beginning of human trials after the ones done on rats is definitely a good start, and shows the potential for CBD. It has been repeatedly demonstrated to reduce inflammation, infection, and balance the endocannabinoid system, all of which can greatly benefit heart health.

CBD is also able to benefit some of the side effects of heart problems, like pain and insomnia. Additionally, it can also be appealing as a treatment since it has no side effects, unlike most modern prescriptions given to those with heart problems.

Despite the current lack of professional research and patient responses based on CBD alone, the testimonies regarding medical marijuana and THC products are promising. One interesting find on a group of patients hospitalized for heart failure found that those who had smoked marijuana consistently before their hospitalization were less likely to die from the complications.

Heart conditions are one of the areas of the body where it is advised to be extra cautious when using CBD oil or other cannabis products. Some researchers believe there may be a possible link from marijuana smoking and strokes, so until more research comes out, it is certainly not a good idea to completely cut off any prescriptions you may be using in favor of CBD, and always consult your doctor if you are considering adding a CBD oil regimen. If you are looking to use CBD to prevent heart conditions, then you are all clear—although until more conclusive proof is out there, don't place too much emphasis on it.

The majority of people who use CBD in hopes of preventing heart disease also use it for its other effects, such as anxiety and general pain relief. Since those doses vary based on weight as well as any other factors you may want to treat, I advise starting small with one dose daily or a few times a week, and increasing if need be.

If nothing else, it can reduce stress and anxiety, which is a leading cause of cardiac arrest and other heart problems, as well as reducing the desire for nicotine, another problem-causing substance in heart health. And of course, keep an eye out as more studies progress, since the medical communities' knowledge of CBD will only continue to grow and expand.

Diabetes

Diabetes is rapidly approaching epidemic levels in the United States alone, with over 100 million Americans living with either Type 1 or Type 2, and another 80 million with pre-diabetes conditions. There is also gestational diabetes, but that only affects pregnant women, and typically disappears after the baby is born.

Diabetes affects the body by causing an imbalance in glucose, or blood sugar levels, usually by making the blood sugar too high for normal functions. This process also involves the pancreas and the hormone insulin, which are what help your body regulate its blood sugar levels. When blood sugar levels in the blood get too high or low, it can cause heart problems, nerve damage, skin conditions, and even comas.

The causes for Type 1 diabetes are still unknown, but medical professionals believe it is a combination of genetic predisposition and environmental factors. For Type 2 diabetes, there is also the chance of genetics and environment, but being obese or overweight can also cause the onset of this disease.

Typical symptoms of diabetes include fatigue, dizziness, being prone to infections, extreme hunger or thirst, and frequent urination. It can happen at any age, even infancy, and is not partial to either gender.

There is no cure for it, only treatment, and the treatments tend to be extremely unpleasant: occasional prescription medications, strict diet restrictions, daily insulin injections, and sometimes even a more permanent insulin pump to help the body regulate blood sugar normally. Patients often have to be taught how to self-administer the insulin shots or injections every day.

It is easy to see, then, how those with diabetes would be hopeful for another type of treatment. Constant injections are not only a hassle to keep up with, but they can be difficult and painful, as well. Another drawback is that taking so much insulin will result in either making it hard to lose weight or gaining a lot of weight.

It is a difficult cycle to break as well as a good motivation to find other alternatives to help you to not be dependent on insulin. Luckily for those with the condition, though, that new research is surfacing pointing towards cannabidiol as a potential treatment.

The current belief is that it may be able to help in a few different ways: first, by preventing the disease altogether, since studies have demonstrated that cannabinoids may be able to lower fasting insulin levels; second, by reducing insulin resistance through its anti-inflammatory effects; and lastly, by aiding the body in treating diabetic neuropathy (nerve damage) and with diabetic related skin conditions.

One study done in 2006 on diabetic rats confirmed this potential. They tested two groups of rats: one that did not receive any CBD treatments, and one that did. They found that the rats who received the CBD treatments reduced their diabetes incidence from 86 percent to 30 percent—an impressive drop. Due to these results, the researchers believe that CBD may be able to slow down problematic insulin issues and accordingly adjust the body's immune system and response.

The study done on the above fasting levels took five years between 2005-2010, and is the only current study done directly investigating the possible link between cannaboids and diabetes. Researchers took a sample of 4,657 adult men and women who were all diabetic, and interviewed each of them individually.

They were asked about their marijuana habits, either at the time or in the past, and then after fasting for nine hours were measured for their fasting insulin, insulin resistance, glucose, and homeostasis. Of the people test, 579 were current marijuana users and 1,975 had used it in the past. Those with a record of marijuana use had, on average, 16 percent lower fasting insulin levels and 17 percent lower insulin resistance than those with no history of marijuana use.

While this study tested traditional marijuana, or weed, instead of CBD, the results of cannabis on diabetes as a whole are absolutely worth paying attention to. This had significant enough results to prompt more studies on cannaboids and diabetes, and hopefully some professional clinical trials, as well.

For those who want to try CBD oil for diabetes and diabetes symptoms treatments, the doses tend to vary based on severity of the condition. And interestingly enough, many actually start with slightly higher doses and then lower them, finding a good consistent daily amount that works for them. For people with more mild diabetes symptoms, an average starting dose is around 40mg per day, dropping back to as little as 10-20mg per day while also monitoring blood sugar levels.

For those with more severe diabetes, people will start as high as 80-100mg per day and then lower it to all the way down to 20-30mg per day. Again, it is important to continue monitoring blood sugar levels, to make sure that the CBD is not negatively interfering with any other medications and is working effectively. These are just starter numbers, and will be affected by other factors such as body weight.

Along with the beginning of clinical studies and research are some impressive stories of patient success. One man reports having diabetes for 25 years, going through an increasingly strict regimen of medications and insulin shots. The amount of insulin then began to increase, as well. He experienced a lot of frustrations, both in dealing with the disease and with the healthcare system that provided treatment.

Finally, he was introduced to CBD oil (supplemented with some THC powder) and after a few weeks of regular dosing, noticed a huge difference. The nerve pain associated with his diabetes was gone, he was sleeping better, and his blood sugar levels were down. He was also able to begin gradually lowering his insulin, and his diabetes 'score' is lower than it had been in years.

Stories such as this one, combined with the evidence supporting the future of more trials should bring a lot of hope to diabetes sufferers. It is almost certain that CBD oil has a place in the diabetic world, and many researchers and patients are simply waiting for the science and medical community to catch up.

Hopefully within a time frame as short as one or two decades we will be able to see a noticeable difference, not only in how diabetes is treated, but also in the amount of people who have it and the severity of their symptoms. 100 million Americans is far too many, and CBD may be just the answer to fix that number.

Chapter 8

Mental Health

There are many physical and bodily diseases helped by CBD, as we have looked at in previous chapters of this book. However, mental illnesses and persistent issues can also be offered relief by these products. There is an ever-growing amount of evidence to support CBD as use against them. Among many of its other benefits, CBD is also known as anxiolytic, which quite literally means it is used to reduce anxiety.

Of the many ailments known to be helped by CBD products, anxiety is one of the more well-known and helped ones. Anxiety disorders cover a spectrum, ranging from Generalized Anxiety Disorder (GAD) to phobia related anxiety, and everything in between. It can affect every aspect of a person's daily life, including work, relationships, and hobbies.

Since it is so widespread and so mentally disabling, it is no wonder people are searching for something simple with fewer side effects than prescription medications such as benzodiazepines, which come with concerns for addiction and other unpleasant side effects.

People get particularly drawn to CBD products for use with this particular problem, since unlike THC products (also known to help anxiety, but with many more variables), there is no risk of getting high. This makes CBD an ideal anti-anxiety product, since it can be used for any circumstance with no worries of intoxication.

Certain CBD products are often exclusively marketed to help with anxiety, in the form of gummies, oil, and for use with vaporizers. There is a surprisingly large, and ever growing amount of evidence demonstrating the effectiveness of CBD to treat anxiety.

Some of said evidence has suggested CBD may be able to help with the brain's production of serotonin, a necessary chemical for normal brain function that tends to lack in people with mental illnesses such as depression and anxiety. Studies are underway to prove this more effectively.

Another mental disorder similar in some ways to anxiety is PTSD, or Post Traumatic Stress Disorder. PTSD is a common response to trauma, and is a common response to time spent in combat or to other traumas such as accidents or sexual abuse. It causes the person to relive the event repeatedly, sometimes for the rest of their life.

Along with anxiety, this can affect all aspects of life, and can be crippling for those who have endured particularly horrible things. It can lead to debilitating anxiety or panic attacks, and PTSD also comes with a depressingly high rate of suicide for its sufferers.

While CBD can't help a person 'get over' PTSD, there is hope that it can alleviate the symptoms and bring relief. The DEA (Drug Enforcement Agency) has recently granted approval for more official studies to begin on the use of CBD to treat PTSD.

Much like the use of CBD for anxiety disorders, CBD can be used to fight the anxiety related effects of

PTSD and bring some relief. It is thought to block the receptors in the brain that can trigger the flashbacks, mood swings, and panic to prevent many of the symptoms from occurring at all.

Insomnia is a common side effect of both anxiety disorders and PTSD, but it is also a problem for many people all on its own. Insomnia is characterized by being unable to fall asleep or stay asleep for consistent periods of time. It is often also associated with depression, poor health, and can be a side effect of a large variety of prescription medications. Being unable to get a proper nights' sleep can result in perpetual mental and physical exhaustion, heightening the effects of other problems such as anxiety and stress in general.

CBD for use with insomnia works much like it does with other stress disorders, allowing the user to relax into sleep and sleep for more prolonged periods of time than they may normally be accustomed to. Since another frequent cause of insomnia can be physical pain, which CBD is also known for helping with, it can serve multiple purposes at once by relieving this pain and helping to increase sleep.

One particular study has gone to show the benefits of CBD against all three of these disorders. In 2015, two medical practitioners tested the use of CBD oil in a young girl who suffered from PTSD due to sexual abuse, and also had anxiety and insomnia issues as a result of this trauma. She had a host of other contributing factors: a history of mental illness in the family, parental deaths, neglect and abandonment.

When she first began trying various treatments (including prescription medications and therapy) she was unable to sleep alone and showed signs of aggression, low self-esteem, and lack of obedience. The CBD oil was not tried until several years after her other initial treatments began and ended. She began CBD oil treatments in March 2015.

At the time, she received a small dose at night (25 mg) to aid with sleep, and she had a CBD spray to use as needed for anxiety throughout the daytime hours. After five months on this, she was not only able to sleep both through the night more consistently and by herself, but she also had a notable increase in daily anxiety and was tolerating school much more effectively than she had previously.

The success of this study lends extremely positive results to the CBD community as a whole. It was able to decrease the negative effects of a myriad of problems in a young girl, greatly increasing her quality of life without any other prescription medications, and no side effects noted by either of the physicians on her case.

Since such small doses, used consistently, were able to cause such a drastic result in a girl with so many traumas, there is certainly an arguable case to be made that similar doses can have the same progressive effects on many other people.

There are hundreds of people across the country and the world who pledge to the benefits of cannabis to treat their anxiety. One man tells of his several years long battle with the mental disorder. He tried a range of prescription medications, none of which were particularly effective.

Like many other people on anxiety treatments, he felt as though they made him groggy and zombie-like. After being completely off medication for a while and continuing to struggle with anxiety, he was recommended CBD oil and decided to try it. After a few false starts, he began dosing regularly and found himself to be more clear-headed, calm, and functional than he had in years.

This story is nearly identical to many others'. CBD can provide wonders for those with anxiety disorders, and some of the most commonly reported strains for this use include Harlequin, ACDC, CBD Shark, and Trident. The average dose varies based on body weight and severity of the anxiety, but many start with doses as small as 20mg daily and report success.

One mistake regarding CBD use for anxiety to be aware of is to keep in mind that CBD can only do so much. It can be a great aid to calm and neutralize feelings and worry, but it cannot get rid of whatever may be causing the problem in the first place; be it mental illness, trauma, or other stressors.

This is mostly important to remember so as not to end up feeling 'let down' by the CBD, since it is not a cure-all. While there is no inherent harm to trying these products if you are suffering from one of these disorders, it is still advised to talk to your physician and be aware of the way it could potentially interact with prescription medications. Use caution, but give it a go—the results may surprise you.

Substance Abuse

Those who suffer from addiction know the pain and destruction it can bring not only to themselves, but also to those around them. Addiction is a rapidly growing epidemic in the United States, with over 20 million Americans reported to battle some form of substance abuse or addiction in 2014.

Those kinds of numbers are both staggering and depressing, for the reason that addiction is so incredibly difficult to treat and to recover from. It effects all ages from teenagers up, men and women, of all races. There are a variety of drugs to be addicted to, as well, each with their own problems: cocaine, heroin, methamphetamines, opioids, and alcohol.

There has been a significant amount of evidence pointing to the fact that one can be genetically predisposed to addiction, and that addiction is a disease. This is still a hotly debated subject among many, but regardless of whether or not your personal beliefs match up with this, it still cannot be disputed that addiction is both life threatening and hard to kick.

It physically rewires the brains reward systems, causing a rush of dopamine (a chemical that provides pleasure) anytime the drug is used over time. The person receives less pleasure from other things they once enjoyed, or even need to survive, such as eating, sex, hobbies, or spending time with loved ones. Because of this, the only thing that may bring a person happiness or comfort after too much drug abuse is the drug itself, and they will often to go any means to achieve it.

Addiction can never be cured, but it can be treated and managed. The most common treatments involve the use of temporary medications to get through withdrawal symptoms, such as antidepressants and benzodiazepines, and then therapeutic work like rehabilitation and AA or NA meetings. Even these are often only partially successful, as it is more of a support to help the sufferer instead of physical help.

CBD may be changing the face of all that, though. New evidence is coming to light that CBD treatments may be able to help prevent relapse in substance abusers, even long after the CBD itself was taken. One such study was completed in March of 2018, and had impressive results. Like many other trials, it was done on rats.

A group of researchers chose rats with histories of alcohol and cocaine use and gave them CBD by rubbing it topically into their skin once a day for a week. During this time, they monitored the rats for stress and drug-seeking behavior with the help of things such as mazes and stress behavior. What they found was that the rats were less impulsive and less dependent on the substances for up to five months after the trial, as well as having lower levels of anxiety.

When placed in stressful situations, the rats were less likely to use substances, and since stress and anxiety are often causes of human relapses as well, this positively demonstrated the use of CBD as both beneficial for reducing the desire to relapse, and for having long term effects with only a small amount of treatment. This is an extremely hopeful study and will hopefully have similar results replicated across more trials.

The potential for a long lasting addiction treatment is unheard of and revolutionary. Any current treatment such as medications can only hope to have short term benefits, and any long term abstinence from drug use is left up to the abuser themselves. Since it is also effective on a variety of substances, like alcohol, opiates, and cocaine, it is even more beneficial, especially to those who may suffer from addiction to more than one particular drug.

This is particularly important and relevant information with the rapid rise of the opioid crisis. Medical marijuana has been demonstrated to help people wean off of opiates before, with the use of both vaping CBD and vaping marijuana itself. Both of these alternatives are safer than other natural products people use in an attempt to kick addiction, such as kratom.

Kratom is also a plant product, a natural stimulant or sedative, depending on the dosage. While it does have its benefits for addiction recovery, it is also an addictive substance itself, which already reduces some of the effect of those benefits. If more trials can be done on CBD, then addicts may truly have a safe alternative on their road to recovery.

CBD is also thought to help people quit smoking cigarettes and reduce tobacco dependency, as well. One such study was listed in Chapter 22 (Case Studies) but that is not the only demonstration of the use of CBD as a method to curb tobacco cravings. A similar one was conducted in 2013, on a group of 24 regular smokers. 12 of them were given CBD for a week, and 12 were given a placebo in a typical double blind test.

The CBD was in the form of an inhaler or vaporizer, and they were instructed to use it anytime they wanted to smoke a cigarette. The smokers who received the placebo showed no change, while those who were inhaling the CBD showed up to a 40 percent drop in smoking over the week, as well as lingering effects after the CBD treatment stopped.

Tobacco use and nicotine addiction is one of the most common in America, although that number has been slowly decreasing in recent years. Cigarette smoking has been around for decades, and due to its full legal status, many are not willing to give it up, and those who try have to struggle with having easy access to them as well.

1 in 6 people smokes, and over 20 percent of recorded deaths in the United States can be attributed to tobacco smoking in some way, whether it be from the actual smoking, cancer, or secondhand smoke problems. It also has a psychological component, since smoking is often a habit formed over many years, and humans are inherently creatures of habit.

While researchers are not quite positive yet how CBD acts on the brain to help with addiction, the speculation is that it functions by working with the reward system to help neutralize it and reduce anxiety, thus lowering the desire and craving for substances. Whatever the science behind it may be, there is no denying it may end up being extremely useful in the near future as a method for addiction treatment.

If you or somebody you know is considering using CBD to try and treat addiction, it may not hurt to attempt it. Even if the least it does is calm anxiety and reduce the desire to return to substances, this can be a small but generous leg up to those in recovery.

As always, talk to the leading doctor on the case, and use caution, as CBD is still a substance and should be used carefully on those with a history of substance abuse. Despite its non-addictive and psychoactive qualities, every recovery road is different, and staying away from any substance altogether may be the best option.

If you do choose to take this route, there are a few strains that people report are particularly helpful with anxieties and substance problems. Harlequin, Cannatonic and CBD Shark are all popular for these.

The doses people typically take for anxiety and other mental effects are higher than those for some physical problems, with ranges anywhere from 40mg to 600mg daily, based on a variety of factors including weight, the substance used, the severity of the treatment, and the levels of anxiety.

Until there is more information out about CBD and its use for this particular problem, err on the side of smaller doses, and work your way up if need be.

Depression is almost an epidemic as of recent years, affecting around 15 million Americans every year. This is over 6 percent of the total population, and is a staggeringly large number of affected. It is the leading cause of suicide, and it can be caused by a range of factors, including genetics, traumas such as loss of a loved one or tragic accidents, substance abuse, side effects from diseases such as cancer, and a range of other triggers. Once someone has it, unfortunately, it is extremely hard to ever fully beat, although it is treatable with therapy, support, and the use of prescription medications.

Many people who suffer from depression, however, do not like said prescription medications. There are often complaints that they can lead to emotional numbness, people worry about addiction and dependency, and frequently when the symptoms start to lessen due to treatment they no longer think they need it, so they will stop taking the medication.

Depression medications are also known to come with a lot of unpleasant side effects, ranging from physical issues such as decreased sexual desire, weight fluctuation, insomnia, and nausea, to mental issues like increased suicidal ideation, strange dreams, and anxiety.

These kinds of side effects can make it easy to see why people would want to turn to more natural remedies such as CBD, and since many people have had relative success using it to treat anxiety, it would make equal sense for it to be beneficial for depression, as well.

Depression affects the brain by inhibiting the output of necessary hormones like serotonin, dopamine, and cortisol. It does this by interacting with three major areas of the brain: the amygdala, the hippocampus, and the prefrontal cortex. Each of these does an important job regulating the human body. The amygdala controls fear and pleasure responses to things, the hippocampus works with memories and cortisol, and the prefrontal cortex is in charge of emotions, new memories, and decision making.

CBD oil is suspected to help with this mental illness by helping the receptor 5-HT1A produce serotonin more effectively. Raising the serotonin levels in your brain assists the hippocampus in its functions, which in turn allow for healthier basic needs like appetite and sex drive. CBD also is thought to stimulate the growth of new neurons, which prevents the brain shrinkage that often comes with depression.

One study was done on rats to determine whether or not CBD actually did interfere with these 5-HT1A receptors. Researchers gave mice either CBD, an antidepressant, or a placebo, and submitted them to either a swimming test or an open field. Some of the mice were also given a 5-HT1A antagonist before receiving the CBD, to see if it would have an additional effect. What they found was that the mice who received the CBD performed better in the swimming test, and that the CBD behaved very similarly to the antidepressant.

These results are fairly promising for the future of CBD as a potential mood stabilizer. Some researchers have also proposed that in major mood disorders like depression and anxiety, the body's endocannabinoid system gets out of balance, and that CBD helps it return to its original state of homeostasis.

By working with both the endocannabinoid system and the 5-HT1A receptors, the CBD can do a sort of double duty to help the body regulate itself and temporarily lessen the effects and symptoms of depression. Sometimes, this can make all the difference.

CBD should not be considered as an alternative to more traditional methods of managing depression, at least not until much more clinical research is done. However, many people have reported its benefits as a method of helping to ease the anxiety and daily moods that are prevalent in this disorder. Vaping is a popular method of ingesting it among those with depression, and many say that when combined with prescription medications, it creates an overall boost that can improve a few days up to a week with regular ingestion.

Schizophrenia is another mental disorder many are hoping can be helped by CBD oil. Psychosis is similar to this in many ways, although psychosis is a symptom of other disorders such as depression, bipolar disorder and schizophrenia, and is not an entire mental illness in itself. With that said, an episode of psychosis can have similar symptoms to schizophrenia.

They are both characterized by 'breaks' from reality, or being unable to tell what is real. This can happen via hallucinations of any of the five senses, paranoia, a lessened interest in reality, and insomnia, among other things.

Like depression, many things can lead into the onset of psychosis. Traumas, mental illness, brain injuries, and other degenerative diseases like Parkinson's or Alzheimer's. And also like depression, psychosis is thought to be affected by the lack of a production of dopamine, which interacts with a neurotransmitter called glutamate. The glutamate levels drop, while the dopamine rises, creating a significant chemical imbalance in the brain.

CBD does not stop psychosis, or prevent the onset of it as a symptom of a larger disorder, but it is believed to be able to help calm the effects and lessen the symptoms. Researchers suspect it reacts to psychosis in similar ways as it does depression, by regulating dopamine production and interacting with the 5-HT1A receptors to normalize the brains hormones.

GW Pharmaceuticals, based out of the UK, did a trial in 2015 to test cannabidiol on schizophrenia. They ran the test on 88 patients, some of whom received the treatment and some of whom received a placebo. All of them were on some sort of anti-psychotic medications already, and did not stop taking them during the time of the trial.

CBD tested to be superior to be placebo consistently throughout the entire test, with very little side effects and none that appeared to interact with the existing anti-psychotic medications. The researchers reported significant improvements on the patients, many of whom were very unreceptive to previous medications. They also believe that this trial is just the first of many to come in the future regarding the use of CBD on psychiatric conditions.

For many people with mental disorders, these sorts of results are extremely promising. At the end of the day, however, depression is ultimately a deeply personal disorder, and how a person chooses to treat it is a personal choice as well.

If you think CBD may be a viable option to help treat your depression or psychotic symptoms, it is worth consulting your doctor and taking a look into.

Even if it only brings mild relief, that can still be the extra push it takes to help get you through the day. As anyone with depression knows, the littlest things can sometimes make all the difference.

Chapter 9

CBD
and animals

While CBD oil is typically thought to be a treatment for humans, there is some potential for it as a pain relief drug for animals, as well. While there is currently not a lot of professional grade research done, some studies are underway during the writing of this book. We will touch on one of the already completed ones in this chapter.

It should be noted that, as with humans, CBD cannot cure any ailments in cats, dogs, or any other pets. It can be used as an attempt to bring relief, or treat symptoms, but should not have too much placed on it if your pet is truly suffering. And as with human use, it is a good idea to consult with a veterinarian before trying it out on your pet, especially if they receive other medications for medical conditions.

Most of the hope for CBD use and animals comes from the use of regular people on their pets through vet recommendations—with slightly mixed results. The parents of these pets have reported easier sleep, less anxiety, and improved appetites and attitudes from their animals.

Some people have also used it on their dogs with cancer who had no other hope for treatments, and reported major improvements in the day to day life of the dogs as well as increased longevity. These were typically extremely small doses—often as small as 0.25 mg per half pound of the dog.

A few things CBD has been thought to improve in dogs include inflammation, heart health, cancers and tumors, bowel issues, anxiety, and seizures. While dogs and humans have quite different genetic makeups, the cannabidiol acts similarly in their systems by neutralizing the endocannabinoid system to promote homeostasis.

This sounds complicated, but in layman's terms essentially means that CBD helps this system from heading towards extremes, and allows it to act and function the way a normal and healthy endocannabinoid system does.

Cats are another common pet that the CBD industry is working on helping. However, caution should be used regarding cats, as cannabis plants themselves are thought to be toxic. It will not kill them, but there are documented cases of pets eating marijuana and becoming sick. Of course, since CBD is *not* marijuana, it typically will not have these effects, but keeping this in mind can only keep your furry friends safer.

For cats, CBD is thought to help with several different anxieties as well as physical ailments. Some of the common cat anxieties include introduction to new cats, litter box problems, consistent crying, and hiding.

And along with dogs, it is thought to ease aches and pains, help with cancers, and reduce inflammations. These cats are also receiving extremely small doses, from 1-5 mg or less. This is typically determined, both in cats and dogs, by the body weight of the animal in question.

One study done recently by Cornell tested the effects of CBD oil on dogs with osteoarthritis. The goal was to see if it could effectively reduce some of the pain and discomfort on these dogs, whose only other options were prescription medications.

Much like many of the studies we have looked at that tested on humans, the researchers had two control groups: some received CBD capsules every 12 hours, for four weeks, and some received placebos for the same amount of time. The results were fairly positive—the dogs who received the CBD treatment showed decreased lameness in their joints over the period of time, while the dogs who received the placebos showed no change.

While this study is promising, few others have yet to come to light. Ultimately, a lot more research is going to have to be conducted on humans before the same treatments will begin to trickle down to our furry friends, but the interest and curiosity is out there, waiting to be tapped into. And if you are interested in trying these products on your pet (with caution!) there are a plethora of products on the internet marketed and branded specifically for cats and dogs.

Do your research on the product and ingredients beforehand, though, and get a vet recommendation if at all possible in your state, as the FDA has reported that many CBD products for pets can have toxic ingredients in them, and sometimes contain no CBD at all depending on the country.

I wish you and your pets the best of luck, and hope that CBD is able to help them with their ailments in similar ways it has helped people over the years!

· Chapter 10 ·

CBD
Recipes

When most people think of marijuana products in food, they typically think of stereotypical foods such as pot brownies. However, the cannabis food community is growing every day—there is even a show on Netflix all about cooking with marijuana. The same thing can easily apply to CBD oil. It is easier to cook into your favorite foods than you think, and here are a few delicious recipes to get you started!

CBD Magic Cookie Bars

This tasty and unique dessert recipe can be stored for up to a week with no worries of getting stale, and will surely be a hit. This recipe takes 15 minutes to prepare, 30 to cook and creates around 20 servings.

What's in it

- 1/4 cup butter
- Condensed milk (14 ounces)
- Caramel chips (0.5 cups)
- Flakes of coconuts (1 cup)

- Preferred kind of nut (1 cup)
- Chocolate chips (1 cup)
- Graham cracker pieces (.8 cups)
- Graham cracker crumbs (1.5 cups)
- CBD Oil (2-3 T)
- Butter (.25 cups)

How it's made

To begin, heat oven to 325 degrees Fahrenheit. Thoroughly spray a 9x13 inch pan for baking, keeping spray evenly coated.

Prepare butter by melting in a small pan. Next, mix your butter, CBD oil and graham cracker crumbs together by stirring.

This should create a mixture resembling a sort of cookie crumble. Press this into the bottom of your pan, adding some larger pieces of graham cracker to the crumble.

Next, spread the condensed milk evenly over the coating of graham crackers.

Pour chocolate chips on the coating, being sure this is even and spread as well. Do not use all your chips yet, some of them will go on top later.

As you do this, also add in the nuts, caramel chips, and coconut. Save a little of each for after it is baked.

Bake this in the oven for 25-30 minutes.

When it is nearly done, take pan from oven and put the rest of your chips, nuts, and coconut on it. Place back in oven for the remainder of cooking time.

Take out of oven and cool. These are best served at room temperature or refrigerated. Enjoy!

Easy CBD Infused Guacamole Dip

For those who want their daily dose of CBD in a more casual way. This recipe takes 20 minutes to make and creates about 4 servings.

What's in it

- 1 Serrano Chile, minced
- ½ diced tomato
- Cut onion (.25 cups)
- Taste of pepper
- Salt (1 tsp)
- CBD oil (1 tsp)

- Lime juice (1 T)
- 2 Avocados

How it's made

Cut avocados in half, removing the pit. Scoop out the insides and put them in a bowl.

Add in the lime juice, CBD oil, salt, and proceed to mash them all together. This can be done with a fork. Be sure to leave it a little chunky

Next, mix in the remaining ingredients: pepper, onion, tomato, and chili

Set in the fridge to cool for one hour. Enjoy!

CBD Infused Spaghetti Sauce

This savory recipe goes great with pasta, and will allow you to get your CBD in a delicious manner. This recipe takes 15 minutes to prepare, 70 minutes to cook and makes about 8 servings.

What's in it

- Sugar (to taste)
- Salt (to taste)

- Onion powder (1 tsp)
- Garlic powder (1 tsp)
- Chopped garlic cloves (2)
- Parsley (1 T)
- Oregano (1 T)
- Sliced mushrooms (1 cup)
- Chopped onion (1)
- CBD oil (2 tsp)
- Tomato sauce (26 oz)
- Tomato puree (26 oz)
- Tomatoes (26 oz)

How it's made

First, mix the tomatoes, tomato puree and tomato sauce together within a big pot. Place this on the stove over low to medium heat and keep covered.

In a different pan on the stove warm up the CBD oil over low heat, then adding in the onion and mushrooms. Mix these together well.

Add salt and pepper to the pan with the CBD oil in it, warming but not browning the onions.

Put your vegetables in the pot with the tomatoes, also adding in the oregano and parsley. Cover and stir occasionally.

Next, once this is all simmering together mix in the garlic and garlic powder and continue stirring occasionally while it simmers.

Put on low heat and allow to continue simmering for an hour.

After this time taste, put in pinches of sugar if too salty or acidic.

Serve, and Enjoy!

CBD Infused Strawberry and Banana Smoothie

A quick, healthy drink treat that can be served at any time of day. This recipe takes 5 minutes to prepare and makes 1-2 servings.

What's in it

- Chopped strawberries (2 cups)
- Chopped fresh banana (1)
- Plain or vanilla yogurt (1 cup)
- Ice (1 cup)
- Honey (1 T)
- CBD oil (.5 tsp)

How it's made

Simply mix everything together in a blender, blend thoroughly, and serve immediately. Enjoy!

CBD Chocolate Chip Cookies

For those with a sweet tooth, this delicious dessert recipe is sure to both satisfy your craving for sugar and get your dose of CBD. This recipe takes about 20-25 minutes to prepare, 15 to cook, and makes about 24 servings.

What's in it

- Chocolate chips (2 cups)
- Flour (3 cups)
- Salt (1 tsp)
- Baking soda (1 tsp)
- Vanilla extract (2 tsp)
- Large eggs (2)
- Sugar (2 cups)
- CBD infused oil (2 oz)
- Butter (1 cup)

How it's made

Ensure your oven is heated to 350 degrees Fahrenheit.

Ensure your butter is softened, and mix it in with the CBD infused oil and sugar and mix it until it is consistently smooth.

Next, mix in the eggs thoroughly and then add vanilla.

In a separate small bowl, mix baking soda and salt with a tiny amount of hot water. Add this to the batter.

Put your flour into the bowl and continue mixing thoroughly. All ingredients should be well blended before adding the chocolate chips.

Continue stirring while mixing in chocolate chips.

Place spoonfuls of dough onto a greased pan or cookie sheet, spaced about two inches apart.

Bake for about 10-15 minutes, cookies should be golden brown around the edges.

Let cool and serve. Enjoy!

For those who may want to apply their CBD instead of ingesting, there are easy ways to make your own products if you would rather not buy them, or live somewhere where that may not be easy. There are a few simple methods for creating a topical CBD treatments:

First, either buy an oil infused with CBD such as coconut, or make your own using Chapter 4.

To make a salve, mix 1 cup of the infused oil and .3 cups of beeswax in a bowl. You can add a few drops of your favorite essential oil here for a nice scent. Heat up the mixture on the stove until it is all melted and blended together. Pour into a bowl, whisk, and let cool until your desired thickness. Then simply add it to a glass storage container!

For a lotion, repeat the above steps, and then mix in aloe vera gel, shea butter, or cocoa butter. Place it in a glass storage container, and you are good to go!

If you would like to work CBD oil into your dog's life, here is a quick and easy recipe to do so. It takes about 15 minutes to prepare, 30 to cook, and makes 30 treats.

What's in it

- Ripe mashed banana (1)
- Peanut butter (.25 cups)
- Whole wheat flour (2 cups)
- CBD infused coconut oil (1 T)

How it's made

Ensure that your oven is preheated to 325 degrees Fahrenheit.

Either grind the oats by hand or place them in a blender until they reach the consistency of flour.

In a separate bowl, mix together the peanut butter, banana, and coconut oil.

Once that is thoroughly mixed, stir in the flour. After it has blended, knead to desired consistency.

Use a small cookie cutter to shape the treats, and place them on a greased or non-stick cookie sheet a couple of inches apart.

Bake in the oven until golden brown for about 30 minutes.

Let cool, store in an airtight container and provide them to your pet when needed!

Some Final Tips for Cooking with CBD

Do not feel limited by the idea that CBD or even cannabis can only be cooked into sweets—there is a whole world of savory options out there as well! CBD will hold its potency better if it is infused into a fat such as butter, coconut oil or lard.

Heat matters! When cooking with CBD, keep it at lower temperatures to prevent evaporation and loss of the cannabinoids. It can also become very bitter if it gets too hot.

Less is more! Do not feel the need to dump extra CBD into your recipes—start small, and if you want more effects increase the dosage gradually.

You will get better results by actually cooking and infusing the CBD into your food than you will if you pour it on top after the food is cooked.

Happy cooking!

Chapter 11

Case studies

As CBD grows increasingly popular, interest from scientists and the medical communities have grown along with it. While there are dozens more clinical trials to be had before anything can become fully approved for prescriptions from a doctor, there have already been some great studies done to really show the benefits of this new wonder oil.

Along with an increase of studies, there is also an influx of people testing CBD out for themselves to get the results firsthand. Some of the stories and success are extremely positive and can be encouraging for those looking to foray into the world of CBD for the first time.

One such study took place in 2011. It aimed to test the ability of CBD oil to help those with Generalized Anxiety Disorder (GAD) to be able to perform public speaking. Public speaking is generally known to be one of the most frightening tasks for anyone with an anxiety disorder, and is actually the top listed fear among Americans in general.

The study was conducted on 24 people, some of which received the CBD treatment and some of which received a placebo instead. None of them had ever gotten any kind of help with their anxiety disorders prior to this test, which can lead to a more 'pure' form of results. The CBD was put into 600mg capsules, and given to the subjects and hour and a half before the test. The subjects were measured for their blood pressure and heart rate, among other things, at six different times during the test.

The results to this were positive for CBD. The subjects who had received the CBD capsules showed far less anxiety and discomfort during their speeches, and also almost completely got rid of negative self-evaluation, which is basically "looking down" upon yourself before any kind of performance, test, or otherwise stressful ordeal, and can have a lasting impact on self-esteem.

The subjects who had received the placebo maintained higher levels of anxiety, discomfort and stress throughout the entire test, effectively demonstrating the potential benefits for CBD against anxiety disorders. This is one of the most well-known and cited cases among the CBD and medical marijuana community in regards to the future of CBD and its future use.

Another study done in the United Kingdom shows encouraging results for those looking to overcome tobacco addiction. It was made up of thirty random smokers, none of whom were under any kind of treatment for their smoking habit at the time of the study. Like the previous study, some of these participants were also given a placebo to test against the real results. They were given either the placebo or 800mg of CBD oil in capsule form, and tested for their reactions to tobacco related stimuli, as well as withdrawals, cravings, and side effects.

After a night of not smoking, researchers compared the results. What they found was that one dose of the CBD reduced the importance of the cigarette cues to the smokers, while those who had received the placebo had no effect. They also reported that CBD did not influence tobacco cravings or withdrawals. Although it had little effect on the actual tobacco addictions themselves, reducing the desire of smokers to smoke was still a notable finding, and one researchers are working on expanding on.

One final case study to review comes from an earlier chapter on the history of CBD. The aforementioned Dr. Raphael Mechoulam, considered the "Father of Marijuana" and the leading cannabinoid researcher in the world, and a group of scientists/researchers from South America compiled together a group of 16 epilepsy sufferers in varying ages (though quite a bit were children) with varying degrees of severity to test the abilities of CBD to stop and prevent seizures.

Since this was one of the very first studies done on humans, they were simply looking to see if the CBD could do this with no severe side effects. They also wanted to see the true effects of CBD on the endocannabinoid system as a whole.

Many of the children tested on suffered as many as 20 to 40 seizures today, and the results were wildly successful: CBD improved every single one of the conditions drastically, with virtually no side effects. Since then, there have been a host of other clinical trials specifically revolving around CBD and epilepsy, and all of them have had great levels of success, as well.

This was considered revolutionary and a breakthrough in the field of medical marijuana, and would help influence laws later such as "Carly's Law" in Alabama, which specifically allows the possession of CBD for epileptic seizures.

Along with clinical trials and case studies, there have been some surveys done among CBD oil users to check in on their satisfaction with the treatment. One general survey done on an extremely large group of users found that not only were over half of the users women, but that the women preferred CBD high strains while men preferred those with THC.

The same study also revealed that the most common ailments people were looking to treat were anxiety, depression, and body pains. Eighty percent of the group said they were extremely happy with the treatment, and over half of them have stopped using other types of medication for their problems altogether.

A few other noteworthy facts from the same survey included that the general consensus agreed cannabis-derived CBD was superior to hemp-derived CBD, and that vaping was the most popular method of taking the product. While these are simply user replies, and not scientifically backed by researchers, these results are nevertheless interesting and extremely positive for the future of cannabis.

Unlike many prescription medications, which typically come with unending lists of side effects and specifications for treatment, nearly all CBD trials have had some level of success. With more trials and research coming out every year, CBD will only continue to push forward as the wonder drug it truly is.

Chapter 12

FAQ's

What exactly is CBD oil?

CBD oil, or cannabidiol, is an extract produced from the Cannabis Sativa plant. CBD itself comes from hemp, which is a slightly different plant then the traditional and more well-known marijuana plant.

Does CBD get you 'high,' like marijuana?

Hemp, which CBD is derived from, only contains trace amounts of THC, which is the actual chemical that gets you high. So no, you cannot get high from any CBD products at all.

Can I fail a drug test from taking CBD products?

Drug tests do not look for CBD, but if the products you are using contain amounts of THC in them, it is possible to fail, although highly unlikely.

Is CBD legal?

CBD has been legalized for medicinal use in almost every state, although it is still not legal on the federal level.

Can I become addicted to CBD?

Due to its lack of psychoactive effects, it doesn't affect the brains reward system associated with other addictive drugs. Even CBD with traces of THC has been shown in studies to have no addictive qualities whatsoever.

How can I ingest CBD?

The most common method is orally; it can be made in food, taken in capsules or as oil, or even in gummies. It can also be put in products like lotion. The quickest way to ingest it, and one of the most popular, is by using a vaporizer.

Is CBD safe to use?

If you are looking to use CBD for health reasons, you should always consult your physician first, but CBD itself is generally known to be a very safe product with few to no negative side effects.

How much does it cost?

This will vary greatly depending on your state, the quantities, and the type of product it is coming in.

Where can I buy CBD?

Along with pricing, this will vary on your state due to legality. The easiest way to find this is to look up your state laws and the best routes to take from there.

Do I need a prescription to get CBD?

You do not need a prescription to get CBD products, depending on your state.

How does CBD work?

CBD is made up of cannabinoids, which react with the endocannabinoid system in the human body. Some evidence has suggested the presence of CBD makes this system produce more of the endocannabinoids, which fight against things like cancer.

Are there any side effects?

While very few side effects have been associated with CBD treatments, a couple have been noted, such as drowsiness, diarrhea, and the potential for shifts in weight or appetite.

What should I look for when purchasing CBD?

There are a few things to make sure of, especially when buying online: that it is organic, that the strain, CBD and THC content are all listed, and that the seller has a good reputation. You can be sure of the last one by checking for reviews.

Will CBD interact with prescription medications?

Depending on the medication being taken, it is possible for CBD oil to have an effect on the enzymes that process that medication.

Chapter 13

Conclusion

Thank you for making it through to the end of *CBD Oil for Pain Relief*, let's hope it was informative and able to provide you with all of the tools you need to achieve your goals involving CBD, whatever they may be.

The next step is to take this new knowledge, and put it towards your own personal use. Whether it be medicinal, for anxiety, or just to broaden your horizons on the cannabis plant, I encourage you to try it for yourself (within reason, of course) and test out its many benefits. My hope is that this book will serve as a guide to you for whatever your use may be, now and in the future.

The cannabis community will naturally continue to progress, and we should strive to progress with it. While it evolves, be sure to stay stringent in your own research so that you can progress with it. As I said previously, it's important to continue to work to destigmatize such a widespread and useful oil that does not deserve the amount of prejudice often placed against it. Every day we can work towards a future with easier access to this wonderful product.

Finally, if you found this book useful in any way, a review on Amazon is always appreciated! I wish you the best of luck in all future endeavors!

Sources

If you would like to look further into your research, or simply want to check out the details of the clinical trials referenced for yourself, you can find them listed below.

"Alzheimer's Controlled With Cannabis At Age 92." *Cannabis Oil Success Stories*, **www.cannabisoilsuccessstories.com/alzheimer-s--92-yo-female.html**.

"CBD for Diabetes - Denny's Story." *CBD School*, 3 July 2018, **www.cbdschool.com/cbd-for-diabetes-part-2/**.

"GW Pharmaceuticals Announces Positive Proof of Concept Data in Schizophrenia." *GW Pharmaceuticals, Plc*, 12 Oct. 2016, **www.gwpharm.com/about-us/news/gw-pharmaceuticals-announces-positive-proof-concept-data-schizophrenia**.

"Patient Success Stories." *#Illegallyhealed*, 26 Dec. 2016, **www.illegallyhealed.com/patient-success-stories/** .

Bergamaschi, Mateus M et al. "Cannabidiol Reduces the Anxiety Induced by Simulated Public Speaking in Treatment-Naïve Social Phobia Patients." *Neuropsychopharmacology* 36.6 (2011): 1219–1226. *PMC*.

Borchardt, Debra. "Survey: Nearly Half Of People Who Use Cannabidiol Products Stop Taking Traditional Medicines." *Forbes*, Forbes Magazine, 3 Aug. 2017, **www.forbes.com/sites/debraborchardt/ 2017/08/02/people-who-use-cannabis-cbd-products-stop-taking-traditional-medicines/#3ba0b3b82817**.

De Filippis, Daniele et al. "Cannabidiol Reduces Intestinal Inflammation through the Control of Neuroimmune Axis." Ed. Silvana Gaetani. *PLoS ONE* 6.12 (2011): e28159. *PMC*.

Hindocha, Chandni, et al. "Cannabidiol Reverses Attentional Bias to Cigarette Cues in a Human Experimental Model of Tobacco Withdrawal." *Addiction*, vol. 113, no. 9, Mar. 2018, pp. 1696–1705., doi:10.1111/add.14243.

Iffland, Kerstin, and Franjo Grotenhermen. "An Update on Safety and Side Effects of Cannabidiol: A Review of Clinical Data and Relevant Animal Studies." *Cannabis and Cannabinoid Research* 2.1 (2017): 139–154. *PMC*.

J., Sirius. "First Clinical Trial with Cannabis for Huntington's Disease Shows Promising Results." *High Times*, High Times, 24 May 2016, **www.hightimes.com/health/cbd/first-clinical-trial-with-cannabis-for-huntingtons-disease-shows-promising-results/** .

Jadoon, Khalid A., Garry D. Tan, and Saoirse E. O'Sullivan. "A Single Dose of Cannabidiol Reduces Blood Pressure in Healthy Volunteers in a

Randomized Crossover Study." *JCI Insight* 2.12 (2017): e93760. *PMC.*

Jankovic, Joseph, and Mary Ann Thenganatt. "Effects of Cannabidiol in the Treatment of Patients with Parkinson's Disease: An Exploratory Double-Blind Trial." *F1000 - Post-Publication Peer Review of the Biomedical Literature*, Feb. 2014, doi:10.3410/f.718883961.793500378.

Lochte, Bryson C. et al. "The Use of Cannabis for Headache Disorders." *Cannabis and Cannabinoid Research* 2.1 (2017): 61–71. *PMC.*

Morgan, Celia J.a., et al. "Cannabidiol Reduces Cigarette Consumption in Tobacco Smokers: Preliminary Findings." *Addictive Behaviors*, vol. 38, no. 9, 2013, pp. 2433–2436., doi:10.1016/j.addbeh.2013.03.011.

Noonan, David. "Marijuana Treatment Reduces Severe Epileptic Seizures." *Scientific American*, 25 May 2017, **www.scientificamerican.com/article/ma**

rijuana-treatment-reduces-severe-epileptic-seizures/.

Parker, Linda A, Erin M Rock, and Cheryl L Limebeer. "Regulation of Nausea and Vomiting by Cannabinoids." *British   Journal   of Pharmacology* 163.7 (2011): 1411–1422. *PMC*.

Penner, Elizabeth A. et al. "The Impact of Marijuana Use on Glucose, Insulin, and Insulin Resistance among US Adults." *The American Journal of Medicine*, vol. 126, no. 7, pp. 583 – 589.

Perucca, Emilio. "Cannabinoids in the Treatment of Epilepsy: Hard Evidence at Last?" *Journal of Epilepsy Research* 7.2 (2017): 61–76. *PMC*.

Philpott, Holly T., Melissa O'Brien, and Jason J. McDougall. "Attenuation of Early Phase Inflammation by Cannabidiol Prevents Pain and Nerve Damage in Rat Osteoarthritis." *Pain* 158.12 (2017): 2442–2451. *PMC*.

Pickering, Elspeth E, et al. "Cannabinoid Effects on Ventilation and Breathlessness: A Pilot Study of Efficacy and Safety." *Chronic Respiratory Disease*, vol. 8, no. 2, 2011, pp. 109–118., doi:10.1177/1479972310391283.

Rudroff, Thorsten, and Jacob Sosnoff. "Cannabidiol to Improve Mobility in People with Multiple Sclerosis." *Frontiers in Neurology* 9 (2018): 183. *PMC*.

Shannon, Scott, and Janet Opila-Lehman. "Effectiveness of Cannabidiol Oil for Pediatric Anxiety and Insomnia as Part of Posttraumatic Stress Disorder: A Case Report." *The Permanente Journal* 20.4 (2016): 108–111. *PMC*.

Walsh, Sarah K et al. "Acute Administration of Cannabidiol *in Vivo* Suppresses Ischaemia-Induced Cardiac Arrhythmias and Reduces Infarct Size When given at Reperfusion." *British Journal of Pharmacology* 160.5 (2010): 1234–1242. *PMC*.

Watt, Georgia, and Tim Karl. "*In Vivo* Evidence for Therapeutic Properties of Cannabidiol (CBD) for Alzheimer's Disease." *Frontiers in Pharmacology* 8 (2017): 20. *PMC*.

Weiss, L., et al. "Cannabidiol Lowers Incidence of Diabetes in Non-Obese Diabetic Mice." *Autoimmunity*, vol. 39, no. 2, 2006, pp. 143–151., doi:10.1080/08916930500356674.

Made in the USA
Las Vegas, NV
25 February 2022

44565792R00108